PRAISE FOR

WISDOM *of the* EARTH, WISDOM *of the* BODY

"Jennifer Raye's guide to integrating the TCM five-element theory with yoga practice offers all of us an invitation to the wise ecology of our body. Her practical, structured guidance and poetic writing encourage the reader to experience evergreen subtlety and nuance in their practice."

—SCOTT BLOSSOM, integrative Ayurvedic practitioner
and licensed acupuncturist

"In *Wisdom of the Earth, Wisdom of the Body*, Jennifer Raye shares with us a beautifully poetic introduction to the principles of Chinese Medicine, Ayurveda, and yoga. Her writing style is warm and inviting, conveying the flow and harmony inherent in the medicine that she's teaching. Even when simplifying complex principles, Jennifer imparts an appreciation for their essence. As a practitioner, this is a book I will enthusiastically share with my patients and suggest to those who are at the beginning and intermediary stages of study in the healing arts. Jennifer provides us with an excellent introduction to the Chinese Five Elements. The message is that *we are the world, we are the cosmos, and our health and integrity are in no way separate from the natural sphere.* Now, as the delicate web of life hangs in the balance, Jennifer's book is medicine for us, and for our times."

—LONNY JARRETT, MAc, author of *Nourishing Destiny*

"A beautifully woven guide that brings together the wisdom of Chinese Medicine and Ayurveda in a way that feels both accessible and profound. I especially appreciated the depth of research and the seasonal and elemental approach. This book provides a rich and practical resource for yoga students seeking deeper balance through the wisdom of Chinese Medicine and Ayurveda."

—BERNIE CLARK, author of *The Complete Guide to Yin Yoga*

WISDOM
of the EARTH,
WISDOM
of the BODY

—

A SEASONAL GUIDE TO CHINESE MEDICINE
AND YOGA FOR BALANCE AND VITALITY

—

JENNIFER RAYE

Foreword by Tias Little

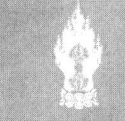

SHAMBHALA

Shambhala Publications, Inc.
2129 13th Street
Boulder, Colorado 80302
www.shambhala.com

Cover art: Elina Li/Shutterstock, VD Igor/Shutterstock, domnitsky/Shutterstock
Cover design: Daniel Urban-Brown
Interior design: Kate E. White

9 8 7 6 5 4 3 2 1

First Edition
Printed in the United States of America

Shambhala Publications makes every effort to print on acid-free, recycled paper.
Shambhala Publications is distributed worldwide by Penguin Random House, Inc.,
and its subsidiaries.

LIBRARY OF CONGRESS CATALOGING-IN-PUBLICATION DATA
Names: Raye, Jennifer author
Title: Wisdom of the Earth, wisdom of the body: a seasonal guide
to Chinese medicine and yoga for balance and vitality / Jennifer Raye.
Description: First edition. | Boulder, Colorado: Shambhala, [2025] |
Includes bibliographical references and index.
Identifiers: LCCN 2025007978 | ISBN 9781645471721 trade paperback
Subjects: LCSH: Holistic medicine | Medicine, Chinese | Yoga | Seasons
Classification: LCC R733 .R39 2025 | DDC 610—dc23/eng/20250609
LC record available at https://lccn.loc.gov/2025007978

The authorized representative in the EU for product safety and compliance is eucomply OÜ,
Pärnu mnt 139b-14, 11317 Tallinn, Estonia, hello@eucompliancepartner.com.

To the most profound and essential teacher,
  this beautiful Earth we call home.
May we wisely honor and revere,
fiercely defend and protect,
and joyously celebrate and nurture
her trees and winds, her waters and soil.

CONTENTS

Autumn Season & Metal Element

Winter Season & Water Element

FOREWORD

The wisdom of the body is immeasurable. As a devoted student of the body, I am in awe of its intelligent, subtle, self-sustaining biorhythms. As a twenty-first-century yogi, what I find most captivating is not only embodiment practices meant to widen my breath, make my spine supple, and clear my mind but also the study of somatic structure, its dynamic function, and its nuanced autonomic rhythms. In the rapidly expanding field of mind-body medicine, *Wisdom of the Earth, Wisdom of the Body* provides key insights into the complex ecosphere of the body landscape.

The farther I travel on the path of practice, studying the nerves, visceral motion, arterial flow, and craniosacral connection, the more I realize that the body is not only immeasurable but ultimately unknowable. No CAT scan, ultrasound, radiograph, or magnetic resonance imaging will ever capture the subtle, all-pervasive force that animates living tissue. For this reason, students of mind-body medicine look to the original Chinese and Indian texts to learn of this invisible force, referred to as Qi and Prana respectively, that prompts every synaptic firing, inspires every arterial pulse, and regulates every heartbeat. Premodern medicine from India and China posited the five elements as the foundation for all physiological activity. However, it was not only Asian disciplines that imagined the body comprised of elements. In fifth-century Greece, Hippocrates, considered to be "the father" of modern medicine, believed the essential biochemical substances to be comprised of four "humors"—water, air, earth, and fire.

In keeping with this spirit of natural medicine, Jennifer Raye brings light and clarity to the practice of embodied wisdom through the synergy of Traditional Chinese Medicine and yoga. When speaking of embodied wisdom, we are referring to the ineffable presence of Prana and

Qi, an imperceptible admixture of energy and spirit. I always find it telling that in the English language there is no word to describe this vivifying force. The best translation we can muster may be "energy," "life force," or "vital air." Embodied wisdom cannot be put down in any formula or prescription. Rather, the wisdom of this medicine is derived from the wind, stars, rivers, and trees. In the Vedas, the earliest scripture from India, it is sourced straight from the gods.

In the way human culture today uses wind farms, solar panel grids, and hydropower stations, practitioners of the internal arts 2,500 years ago tapped the potency of nature to enhance their biorhythms. Yogis and Daoist masters performed their routines in the shade of the forest grove or on the bank of the rushing river. In the Indian Vedas, the gods are wrought from nature's raw forces—wind, fire, lightning, and sky. Consciousness and breath are born from the elements, and postural yoga aims to harness internal wind (*vayu*) and channel internal waterways (*nadis*). The elements are built into the totemic power of animals, and thus many yoga postures incorporate forms within the animal kingdom, including reptiles, fish, birds, insects, and mammals.

It is medicinal to spend time under the open sky in places where the atmosphere is raw and the land uncultivated. As the poet Gary Snyder said, "Good soil is good because of the wilderness in it." Practitioners of the healing arts know, too, that there is a kind of wilderness in the blood, bones, and gut microbiome. When standing on your head or receiving acupuncture for your kidney and liver channels, you are amplifying Prana and Qi. This is the basis for all healing and longevity.

Where I live in the high desert of Santa Fe, New Mexico, I take refuge in remote sandstone canyons. When the wind drops and silence swallows me into its vast presence, I feel a kind of communion with the vital forces all around. I take company in whiptail lizards, nighthawks, and mountain mahogany. Solitude guides me deep inside to a place beyond the configuration of any language. But going off-grid, miles from the nearest traffic light, is not a prerequisite to experience this kind of inner communion. Rather, smack-dab in the middle of your apartment, you need only roll out your mat or sit on your meditation cushion to travel the rivers of your bloodstream, soar on the wind of your breath, and sit solid as granite in your bones. Mostly, you need to be patient, humble, and receptive, open to the wondrous presence of the infinite.

When you enter the temple ground of your body, you come into the presence of something that has existed since time immemorial. For me, the practice leads not to mastery but to a communion with mystery. When I enter the sanctuary of my body, it is like encountering an animal in the wild. Always and foremost, I approach with courtesy, honor, and respect. Ultimately, the internal mechanism—whatever that is—that regulates the nervous system, balances glucose levels, and guides hormonal activity toward homeostasis deserves our greatest awe.

We each inherit a wakeful presence as old as the coelacanth, the horseshoe crab, and the stars. Magnificent, invisible, prevalent as air, it holds us together just as the force of gravity weighs down bone. Every nerve synapse, every fiber of skin, every cell in the body orients to its invisible pull. It is as if a global positioning system has been installed deep inside, from which every heartbeat, every pulse finds its bearing. It is necessary to remember that it is not "you" guiding but the presence of an enormous thing—older, stranger, and wiser than your time-bound self. Every breath and every sensation is linked to the "mind" of this inner navigation. In following its direction, we walk the road of the ancestors. Whether doing a Sun Salutation or Cobra Pose, receiving acupuncture treatment, or retaining the inhalation in pranayama, we align with the potency of this primordial force.

Throughout the pages of *Wisdom of the Earth, Wisdom of the Body*, Jennifer speaks to the profound synergy of body, mind, and vital Qi. She provides new ways of seeing, sensing, and experiencing on the path to embodied wisdom. The bioenergetics of healing in both yoga and Chinese Medicine seep through these pages. This weave of TCM and yoga is timely, as it prompts us to reorient to the natural laws that govern all growth and becoming. I know this weave will bring much vitality, radiance, and clarity to your practice.

—Tias Little
April 2025
Santa Fe, New Mexico

WISDOM *of the* EARTH,
WISDOM *of the* BODY

INTRODUCTION

You Are Nature

If only I had the tiniest grain of wisdom, I should walk in
the Tao, And my only fear would be to stray from it.[1]
—DAO DE JING

Winter has arrived here in the mountains. The autumn larch, like tall golden pillars, have finally given way to big, soft snowflakes, and the sky seems to stretch forever into gradients of blue and gray, bleeding into the horizon. Everything seems at peace in the world, covered in a dusting of glittering white, at least for this moment. In Daoism (one of the primary traditions underpinning Traditional Chinese Medicine, or TCM), winter is the time of year that displays characteristics similar to water. Water is the most Yin of all elemental qualities according to this system, meaning it is darker and colder, just like the season of night and snow. I used to really dislike winter. The cold, dry climate made me long for warmer, more tropical places. But while I still enjoy a good vacation in a warm climate, I've also come to understand that, like all of nature's expressions, winter's retreat and cocooning have their place.

The wisdom of holistic and earth-based medical systems teaches us that each season is simply an expression or pattern of energy. These patterns exist not only externally in the changing sky and trees, but also internally in our bodies and minds. At the heart of traditions like TCM and Ayurveda (the holistic medical system of India and the sister science of yoga) is the recognition that humans are not separate from nature or merely a reflection of nature—we *are* nature. The plants and trees around us create the oxygen we breathe, the earth's minerals fill our bones, and we are made from the water of our planet's oceans. The ancient Chinese Daoists and Indian yogis saw that our bodies and psyches are inextricably bound to an interrelated web of interactions and relationships and are an integral part of the living world. The body-mind is, in fact, a microcosm of the natural world, and nature is a macrocosm of each of us.

By closely observing the rhythms of nature, ancient yogis, sages, seers, and physicians discovered they could develop self-understanding and create states of balance and harmony in their bodies, minds, and spirits. The intelligence of nature exists in every stone, stream, ray of sunlight, and gust of wind. The ancients found that natural patterns affect the budding trees and the nesting birds just the same as they affect us. Nature is teaching us about ourselves all the time if we listen. Natural laws govern our breath and blood and the movement of our minds. They determine the tides of the oceans; the change of light in the sky; and the rise and fall of our energy levels, our moods, and even our capacity for spiritual connection.

Maybe you've encountered some of the earth-based language in these systems. For instance, if you've ever visited a TCM or Ayurvedic doctor, they likely used the language of nature, imagery, and metaphor, along with more recognizable medical terminology, to describe your condition. These systems use words like *cold, damp, wood,* and *water* to describe specific signs or symptoms. For instance, when we experience red-hot inflammation, we use cooling remedies to clear Heat. In TCM, we speak of Wind traveling through the tissues when there are tremors or convulsions, and we understand that an exacting and precise personality is characteristic of the Metal element. In Ayurveda, a person who feels heavy or dull might have too much Earth and Water and need more Fire.

Even though these concepts may sound exotic or esoteric, they describe genuine changes and attributes and are no less tangible or accurate than biomedical terms. They simply depend on perceiving the body-mind as interconnected with more significant natural trends. In these Eastern systems, there is no distinction between life, medicine, and nature. To find health and radiant vitality, we must nurture balance and harmonious flow. This is one of the reasons why Daoism, TCM, Ayurveda, and yoga work so well together. At a basic level, they rely on a similar philosophy of creating balance, and they use the ever-present language of nature to describe patterns of well-being and disease. These ancient wisdom traditions teach us that we can identify natural trends present in the body-mind based on the laws of nature and, therefore, address the root cause of our dis-ease. From there, we can work with diet, lifestyle, therapeutic treatments, and self-care practices to suit our unique needs.

Sometimes patterns of imbalance are apparent, and sometimes they are much subtler. In this way, earth-based systems are both straightforward and complex. This book doesn't attempt to fully explain more nuanced theories. Instead, it aims to highlight how these theories come alive when you start to identify and connect to the energetic properties in nature and your body and mind. These systems have much to offer that anyone can easily and practically apply to their daily lives.

THE RELATIONSHIP BETWEEN CHINESE MEDICINE AND AYURVEDA

Chinese medicine and Ayurveda are two of the oldest and most refined, continuously recorded and practiced healing systems in the world. With thousands of years of testing, trial and error, and rigorous debate among physicians and academics, these elegant and nuanced healing arts have survived and thrived because of their usefulness, accessibility, and efficacy. They also continue to evolve. I see this frequently with my colleagues dedicated to research in the West, and it was especially apparent when I had the privilege of interning at a large university hospital in northeastern China many years ago. There, I discovered how modern TCM doctors are combining Western and Eastern treatments to create an entirely new system of medicine. It was common for patients there to receive both pharmaceuticals and herbal medicines, along with acupuncture and other adjunctive treatments, as a part of their prescription.

Ayurveda and Chinese medicine began independently, and their foundational theories arose from their respective cultures. The philosophies of Daoism and Confucianism heavily influenced the theories of

TCM, which has remained associated with Chinese culture and religious beliefs throughout its evolution. On the other hand, Ayurveda is rooted in Indian sciences and was created from a combination of Sankhya philosophy and various spiritual systems of yoga. That being said, there is significant evidence that practitioners of TCM, Ayurveda, and yoga exchanged information and influenced one another throughout much of history. Early voyages and travel along the Silk Road facilitated and encouraged this sharing of information between spiritual seekers, teachers, physicians, and leaders. At the same time, Buddhist practice and theory originated in India and spread across Japan, Tibet, Sri Lanka, Southeast Asia, and China. This expansion of Buddhism throughout the region further aided the movement and intermingling of ideas, theories, and medical practices. Eventually, this exchange slowed for various reasons, but only after the interweaving of many aspects of TCM, yoga, Ayurveda, and Buddhism.

Personally, I'm grateful to have almost always intertwined the study and practice of these traditions. As a young adult, I explored many holistic modalities and healing arts. TCM, Ayurveda, yoga, Buddhism, healing foods, and Western herbalism captured my attention and set me on my life path. It wasn't long before I found myself knee-deep in textbooks, working toward a doctorate in TCM while at the same time sneaking away to practice and study yoga and Buddhism whenever I got the chance. In the classroom, I investigated the fascinating world of meridians, Qi (pronounced "chee"), acupuncture, and herbal medicine. On the yoga mat, I settled into long silent retreats, somatic exploration, and therapeutic movement. It was the perfect blend for me: the holistic models of Ayurveda, yoga, and Chinese medicine so precisely and beautifully describe what many people encounter and feel while practicing somatic movement, yoga, and meditation—the mystery of the body-mind, a feeling of energetic healing, and the deep interconnection of all things.

Sometimes, I get the question "Why combine TCM and yoga when yoga already has a medical system in Ayurveda?" I've found that even though each framework is a product of its individual culture and a powerhouse of wisdom on its own, they work really well synergistically. They do have their differences, but at their very foundation, they complement each other beautifully. In this book, I attempt to share insights on how to apply this rich mix of traditions to movement, meditation practice, and everyday life while staying true to the integrity of each worldview.

In many ways, all of these traditions constellate around self-exploration, investigation, and understanding to develop higher consciousness, insight, and awareness. They are doorways into sensing, feeling, and working with our internal states and lived experience. They also foster a strong sense of responsibility for, and reciprocity with, the earth and all beings. In myriad ways, we live in a troubled world. Spurred on by many factors, including systems of oppression, domination, and trauma, modern people are often disconnected—from themselves, each other, and the natural world. I believe the momentous task of addressing our social and environmental crisis cannot be fully realized without also addressing this separation. While conventional modern medicine provides profound insight into the structure and function of the body, it falls short in addressing this growing disconnection.

We must start turning toward earth-based medical systems with long and established histories for solutions and support. Our bodies, our minds, and the planet need a paradigm that includes the healing power of earth-based medicine and mindful movement—one that helps us feel and understand our body-mind as interconnected with larger natural rhythms and fosters a deep sense of presence and embodiment. Our bodies move at the rhythm of the earth and in sync with natural laws. It only makes sense then to reclaim natural rhythms and holistic models to truly restore our separation. By strengthening and nourishing our physicality, balancing and vitalizing our subtle energetic system, stabilizing our mind, illuminating our spiritual path, and encouraging us to stay compassionate and courageous, these traditions remind us we are connected to the whole and offer us a kind of homecoming to something greater. They are a refuge we can return to when we are troubled, weary, or lost. In this way, earth-based systems of healing facilitate a deeper relationship with all of life and assist in the healing of the planet.

All these traditions invite us into a place of openness and awe; indeed, they are potent medicine for our times. In the eyes of the ancient sages, seers, yogis, and physicians, the body, mind, and whole universe hold immeasurable wonder and spiritual mystery. Whether it's the concept of the natural elements of fire, earth, or water moving through our blood and bones or visualizing emotions living in our organs, imagery and symbols help us shake loose our rigid understanding of the material realm and see things in a new light. Viewing things in this subtle way helps us access the part of our being that is capable of experiencing spaciousness, freshness, and curiosity. When we're able to tune in to and trust this openness, we can more easily drop our illusion of control and see beyond what is habitual to the very flow of life itself—what Daoists call the Way, or Dao (also written as *Tao*).

WHAT IS THE DAO?

Dao is a rich word with profound meaning that escapes an exact English translation. Everything in the material world we experience is exceptional because it's infused with potential energy from the Dao. Referring to a path or route, the concept of Dao captures both emptiness and fullness and is similar to the quality of oneness, harmony, unity, or wholeness. The Dao is simply the way things are or the natural course of the universe. Every weather pattern, email, thought, traffic light, experience, or sensation expresses this movement of the Dao. It represents an all-inclusive stream, an amazing arising of the present moment, and is just like water—powerful yet yielding, self-replenishing and ever-moving.

The first lines of the classic Daoist text, the *Dao De Jing* (also written as *Tao Te Ching*), point to this unnameable force: "The tao that can be told is not the eternal Tao. The name that can be named is not the eternal Name."[2] In Daoist philosophy, creation begins with this mysterious central organizing principle, and from this untouchable first principle, the polarities of Yin and Yang arise. Then, Qi emerges from the tension between Yin and Yang, further expressing the Five Elements. The Dao is void and unchanging but gives rise to all forms and patterns. Every friendship, fungi, work of art, delicious meal, and stunning landscape is an expression of the Dao.

While the Dao remains a little out of perceptual grasp, there is a way to see it. The diversity of expression in manifest reality reflects its creativity and variability. The Dao can be experienced through the ever-changing lunar and solar cycles, in the cold breeze of a winter night, in the warm soil of a newly dug garden bed, in the deep feeling of lost love or unbearable grief. The philosopher Lao Tzu says, "Open yourself to the Tao, then trust your natural responses, and everything will fall into place."[3]

Interestingly, we don't often question the natural laws that dictate the moon's cycles, the growth of the great cedars, or the seasons' ebb and flow. However, modern people have more difficulty recognizing these same patterns in themselves. "Water draws us closer to the Dao," reflected Lao Tzu nearly twenty-five hundred years ago. The ancients knew we were part of a larger pattern—the great unfolding of the Dao and the rhythm of nature and time. If we move against these natural currents, we will become unwell. To foster health, promote vitality, and avoid disease, we must find our place in nature and learn to move harmoniously with the ever-changing currents of the earth. Even though we share common characteristics, we are still separate from the wisp of cloud, the flowing river, the snowy peak, and one another; we each have a unique path to express in this life. Our multiplicity keeps the intelligent system of our cosmos functional.

So to be in the Dao means to be in the natural and harmonious stream of life. Dao also describes an all-encompassing primordial source that imbues all things with a unique nature, power, or virtue (*de*). The Chinese classics tell us that when we're in balance and following the course of natural rhythms, we have access to a vital or brilliant power (*ming de*) and the capacity for spiritual brightness or awareness (*shen ming*). At a fundamental level, a disconnection from this awareness feeds many states of imbalance in our bodies and minds. However, we each have a part of us that is open and awake that we can access. When we're following our unique Dao in alignment with the Dao of nature, we can work with and potentially heal our physical or mental states and spiritual selves. The essential question and practice then become "How can I live my life following the natural and harmonious pattern, or Dao? How can I honor the expression of Dao and learn to flow with it in every moment?" I look forward to exploring these questions and more with you throughout this book.

HOW TO USE THIS BOOK

I envision this book as a journey of self-discovery and self-awareness. The wisdom traditions and embodiment practices I draw on for this exploration offer a sophisticated and potent way into our bodies, minds, and hearts and give us varied and abundant language to describe and understand what we discover.

When we thoughtfully weave together these traditions, we have access to many techniques—yoga postures, breath practices, acupressure points, meditations, and more—to support us in sensitively perceiving and responding to our inner and outer environment. This can help us live more balanced, connected, and joyful lives. Addressing our imbalances and disconnection also helps us be more available to act with fierce resolve and a wide-open heart on behalf of our troubled world.

This book has two parts. We begin in Part One with some core theoretical concepts. This is where you'll learn some basic TCM language and how to start identifying states of imbalance through self-investigation. We'll look at how the ancients mapped the physical and subtle body, emotions, and spirit, and we'll go over some of the key practices we can use to create embodied health and wellness.

Part Two is where we enter the realm of the Five Elements. It is here that we pair Chinese medicine and Daoist imagery with yoga and meditation practices to create a nuanced system of healing. Although the elements are interdependent—meaning they exist and are developed simultaneously—we will begin with the Wood element and then work our way around the circle of the Five Elements, eventually concluding with Water.

Each element in Part Two has three chapters. The first chapter of each element delves into an explanation of the overall energy, including seasonal self-care, kitchen remedies, physical attributes in the body, and an investigation of the energetic organs and meridians associated with the element. The second chapter covers some key ways we typically go out of balance and some habits and practices like yoga, sense-organ care, breath work, and meditations to help us return to harmony. The final chapter for each element investigates the emotional and spiritual sphere. We'll look at how specific states of consciousness related to each element can be transformed into positive virtues that serve not only us but the greater whole and practices to accomplish this.

It is my hope that this book will aid you in developing a greater capacity to tune in to the subtle (and sometimes not-so-subtle!) natural rhythms of your body-mind for greater vitality and balance. Equipped with this knowledge, you might base your next yoga practice on one of the elements by weaving together movement, acupressure, personal inquiry, meditation and visualization inspired by the natural world—all sitting on a foundation of embodied understanding. Plus, after working on your yoga mat or meditation cushion with the practices and personal reflections, you can apply your insights off the yoga mat too. You don't need to understand everything in this book to use it, although over time I'm certain new layers of understanding will reveal themselves to you.

I hope that you enjoy this book, from my heart (and home) to yours, and that you return to it as a resource and inspiration for many years to come. I also have some resources that go along with the book at wisdomofthebodybook.com. Please feel free to visit my home on the web to explore more.

A NOTE ABOUT LANGUAGE

Throughout this book, you may notice I use three terms interchangeably: *Traditional Chinese Medicine*, *Chinese medicine*, and *TCM*. While many practices and theories in this system derive from ancient texts, it's important to note that it's not necessary to add the word *traditional*. This is because Chinese medicine is not fixed and stuck in the past. It is an evolving system of medicine that continues to grow from its ancient roots. It's now used across the globe, *and* it continues to advance. For this reason, I often refer to the theories in this system as Chinese medicine or TCM.

Please also note that many foundational TCM concepts have roots in the ancient philosophies of Daoism and Confucianism; for this reason and the purposes of this book, I often use the terms *Chinese medicine* and *Daoism* interchangeably when speaking of related theories. Similarly, I occasionally use the terms *Ayurveda* and *yoga* in a comparable fashion.

One of the most common ways people get hung up when trying to grasp the Chinese medicine worldview is not understanding that some translated words have very different meanings in English than in Chinese medicine. For instance, when speaking of a single organ in Chinese medicine, we are referring to an entire system—a whole variety of interactions, processes, and functions not recognized in the West. Therefore, you'll find these special words capitalized to differentiate them from the conventional medical understanding of the word. For example, when speaking of the Chinese medicine substance called Blood or the TCM organ we call Liver, the word is capitalized to differentiate it from what we know as "blood" and "liver" in Western medicine—and to highlight its special meaning. There are also a few Chinese medicine terms I have chosen not to translate as there are no adequate English words to describe the concept. For those untranslated words, I have either adopted the most accepted conventional spelling or referred to the romanization called Pinyin. For herbal medicines, I have included the Pinyin name for remedies generally used in TCM practice and the English name for herbs commonly used in the West.

Finally, the languages of yoga and Buddhism are primarily written in Sanskrit and Pali, respectively. In this book, I only use the Sanskrit language when referring to yoga and Buddhist teachings and have eliminated diacritical marks to minimize any confusion.

SUGGESTED SUPPORT

Today, Chinese medicine and yoga are gaining massive popularity in the West. From their ancient roots to their modern expression, these systems have so much to offer us. They give us a method for looking at the body, disease, and health holistically and can help us take care of ourselves and our communities. As you explore the material in this book, I strongly encourage you to work with a licensed Chinese medicine practitioner and a qualified yoga and meditation teacher to deepen your study and understanding. Especially if you are experiencing health troubles, working with a good practitioner will help you access the depth of knowledge and wisdom these complex healing systems offer. This book is meant to aid in your healing and learning journey and does not replace the advice of your primary health care provider or the wise guidance of a Chinese medicine practitioner. I also encourage you to visit my website at jenniferraye.com and the book's website at wisdomofthebodybook.com for more information and resources.

PART ONE

CORE CONCEPTS

ONE

OUR SUBTLE BODY

Truly, it is prana that shines forth in all things!
Understanding this, one becomes a knower.
—MUNDAKA-UPANISHAD

For many thousands of years, Chinese and Indian yogis have worked with an animating power or energy called Qi in Daoism and Chinese medicine, or *Prana* in Ayurveda and yoga. This potential energy and essential life force exists as a creative field or force that moves everything around and in us. It exists all the way from the outer reaches of space down to the smallest parts of our cells. In the body and mind, it takes endless forms: it lives in our skin, runs through our muscles and spinal fluid, energizes our gastric juices, and inspires our thoughts. It is this life force that determines your levels of vitality, quality of presence, and vivacity of spirit. Every clever idea you have, every muscle twitch you feel, and every heartbeat you sense is Qi functioning and moving.

This is also the inherent energy we experience in the natural world. Our beautiful planet is alive with this vital principle. From the most minute amoeba to the grandest mountain range, Qi expresses itself, moving and transforming in our living animate world. When we sense and enjoy energy outside ourselves, what we're feeling is how Qi binds us inextricably to everything else. It is what connects us to the butterflies and trees and what creates harmony, oneness, or wholeness in all things. I certainly experience this sense of connection and life force when sitting with the breathing ferns and cedars in the dense forest beyond my home.

The Chinese character for Qi shows steam rising from rice, pointing to how it is both intangible, like the vapor rising upward, and full of substance like the grains of rice. All life has Qi, which is both material and immaterial, form and function. The concept of Qi can be challenging to understand because we can't quantify it with scientific measurements; it has no weight, and we can't see it. It eludes our grasp as it is ever-changing and exists only as a state of life. As Qi condenses, it forms structures like our bones and the fibrous stalks of plants. As it disperses, it creates movement, causing synapses to fire, blood to circulate, and the swoosh of wind through the trees.

When we're healthy, our Qi is plentiful, clear, and fluid like a pure watercourse; it flows naturally and easily. It is not dried up, stagnant, or murky. The ancient sages learned to protect, build, harness, and manipulate the distribution of Qi to ensure good and abundant flow in their bodies and minds—and, therefore, health and balance. Chinese and Indian yogis knew that how much energy you start with, how you use it, and how you replenish it during your life determines how well you are and how easily you walk your path in this life. The *Nei Jing* says it this way: "Blood and Qi, [they are] the spirit of man; it is essential to nourish them carefully."[4]

The key is in tapping into and cultivating this creative and eternal source that exists everywhere. The *Dao De Jing* says, "[T]hat is why the sage can act without effort and teach without words, nurture things without possessing them, and accomplish things without expecting merit: only one who makes no attempt to possess it cannot lose it."[5] Essentially, if we live our lives in concert with the amount of Qi we have, we will find our way and be able to express our life's purpose. The good news is that we can consciously cultivate plentiful and flexible Qi through our daily actions, choices, and practices, which we explore throughout this book.

SOURCES OF QI

We get our Qi from two main sources. The first is our prenatal, constitutional, or original (*Yuan*) Qi. The second is our postnatal or acquired

Qi, which we receive from nutrition in food, fluids, and vitality in the air we breathe. These eventually combine to form nutritive (*Ying*) Qi, which circulates in the subtle energetic meridians of the body, nourishing all our tissues and organs.

The first type—our constitutional Qi—is mostly predetermined. The potency and quality of this inborn energy depend on the energy or "essence" we receive from our parents and the nourishment we gain in the womb. This Qi is the genetic blueprint we're given at birth. In Daoism, this links to the idea of de, the innate power or destiny we each hold within. Prenatal Qi is what primarily determines our overall tendencies, strengths, and weaknesses. Ancient Chinese and Indian yogis were particularly focused on protecting this vital life force for purposes of longevity.

It is because of our unique characteristics from our prenatal Qi that we each need different practices and therapies to stay well. For instance, whereas one person may need methods that target stagnant Qi or invigorate energy in a specific system, another may need practices that restore or replenish it. This is based on the inherited energy they were each given at birth. Since this Qi is hereditary, its fundamental strength and characteristics won't change much throughout our lives. However, we can protect, augment, or deplete it based on our chosen life path.

The second type—our acquired Qi—comes from the food and fluids we digest and assimilate and the air we breathe. Food nourishes every tissue and substance in our bodies, and the types of food we choose to eat, how we prepare and combine foods, how we relate to food, and whom we eat it with all determine the quality of acquired Qi we end up with. When we breathe, we take in air, which also contributes to our acquired Qi, affecting every cell within us and influencing our minds. So it's imperative to include fresh air in your self-care practices, such as going for a daily walk somewhere out in nature, especially if you spend a lot of time indoors or in a polluted environment.

QI BALANCE AND IMBALANCE

Qi is the underlying force for all substances and functions in your body. It transports materials like hormones and bile; it holds things where they should be, like keeping blood in your arteries and veins and your organs in place; it transforms substances like food during digestion; it warms you through temperature regulation; and it even protects you from external pathogens like harmful bacteria or viruses. When our Qi is healthy, its amount, quality, and movement are harmonious. It feeds all our tissues, systems, organs, and subtle channels with life-giving sustenance, and the body-mind maintains perfect homeostasis.

When out of balance, our Qi cannot do its good work, and we suffer. For instance, Qi can be rebellious and move in the wrong direction, causing hiccups or heartburn, or it can collapse, leading to a severe organ prolapse. Our Qi can also be deficient, in which case there is too little energy, and our systems, organs, or bodily substances may be inadequate or underactive. For example, if you live a fast-paced life on very little sleep and poor eating habits, your body won't get the energy it needs, and you'll most likely start to have signs of Qi deficiency, such as weak muscles, fatigue, a weak voice, or pale skin. In that case, practices and remedies that build and restore your body-mind are best.

On the other hand, if you have excess Qi, there is too much. This can occur in two main ways. You may have an overactive system (for example, too much blood circulation from drinking alcohol, causing your face to turn red), or you may have a stagnation of some sort. For example, when you get a bruise, blood stagnates in one area and doesn't circulate well. Or, in the case of edema, fluid accumulates where it shouldn't. Another example is developing Qi stagnation in your stomach due to overeating. In these cases, we use methods that either increase circulation or reduce what has become excessive.

In each of these examples, there is an imbalance of Qi. To achieve good health, we need to reestablish the balance and good flow of this life-giving energy.

INNER STOREHOUSES OF QI

Our Vital Organs and Substances

In Daoism and the Chinese medical tradition, our internal organs are not simply masses of tissue. They are powerful expressions of Qi and are alive with energy, spirit, and wisdom. They also act as reservoirs for our Vital Substances—our Qi, Blood, *Jing*, *Shen*, and Body Fluids. The most important of these substances are the Three Treasures—the Jing, Qi, and Shen—we'll explore these in more detail in Part Two. In Ayurveda, *Ojas* has many similarities to Jing, Prana correlates clearly with Qi, and *Tejas* can be matched loosely with Shen. It is these substances that create the seven tissues (*dhatus*) of the body. In TCM, all the Vital Substances, including the Three Treasures, play a role in the creation and function of our tissues and organs. In both Daoist and yogic practices, we need these substances in adequate quantity and quality to achieve physical, mental, energetic, and spiritual goals.

Just as Qi has innumerable expressions in nature, each of your organs and Vital Substances has distinctive physical, energetic, emotional, and spiritual traits. In my medical practice, I look to each of the organs and these fundamental substances to understand a person's overall well-being. In some cases, our energetic organs have similar responsibilities to those of their Western anatomical counterparts. However, they also have many duties and relationships that set them apart. For this reason, we capitalize the names of organs in TCM.

Your organs are grouped as complementary pairs, meaning one has more nourishing "Yin-like" qualities, while the other has more dynamic "Yang-like" qualities. Yin organs are called *Zang*—they are the Lung, Spleen, Heart, Kidney, Liver, and Pericardium. They store Vital Substances and are considered deeper, more solid, and more critical than Yang organs. Yang organs are called *Fu*—they are the Large Intestine, Stomach, Small Intestine, Urinary Bladder, Gallbladder, and *San Jiao*. They constantly fill and empty, taking in food and drink and transforming them to be stored by the Yin organs. They also excrete waste. While each organ in a pair may take a more supportive (Yin) or active (Yang) role, they each still have qualities of both Yin and Yang, nurturance and activity, within them. Our energetic organs also correspond to a natural phase or elemental energy from the Five Element model, which we explore in the next chapter and throughout Part Two.

Once we understand the unique attributes of our energetic organs and Vital Substances, we can begin to develop an inner relationship with them. When we determine they're out of balance, we can harmonize their essential functions and relationships by nurturing their energies through specific self-care tools. For instance, once I understand that my energetic Liver helps to move Qi, its associated sense organ and substance are the eyes and Blood, and the emotion related to it is anger (as we'll explore in later chapters), I'm able to specifically target my practices toward my Liver when I'm experiencing itchy red eyes and a tendency toward frustration.

To sense which type of practice or method might be appropriate, we just need to slow down and tune in. Because Qi permeates our body-mind, it is always communicating its wisdom. Through a vast network of intuitive signals, your body-mind will tell you what it needs on any particular day. I refer to this as "attending" because we need not do anything too special. Instead, our inner world simply requires time and space to show itself. In Part Two, we'll explore some specific ways to listen internally to the Qi of the body and vital organs.

Our Subtle Body Network

One of the most remarkable similarities between Chinese medicine and yoga is that they recognize we have both a physical structure and a finer, more delicate, subtle body. We contain an elaborate and intelligent system of energetic pathways, pressure points, animating currents, and subtle centers where Qi moves and collects. While they don't have an exact physiological equivalent, these radiant centers, channels, and energy flows have more refined and gross facets. They influence aspects of the mind and spirit just as they affect states of health and disease in the body.

While the ancients may not have charted our physical anatomy with much detail (mostly because of the ideas prominent at the time regarding dissection and the sanctity of the body), they did describe a very complex network of energetic pathways. The energy, or Qi, we explored earlier not only dwells in your organs and circulates your Vital Substances, it also flows through this invisible and intricate system of channels.

Both Chinese and Indian traditions maintain that the elegant mapping of our subtle body emerged out of the insights ancient sages had during deep states of meditation and contemplation. In Ayurveda and yoga, channels are called *nadis* and *srotamsi* (or *srota*). Srota are more physical and functional, while nadis are subtler. In Sanskrit, the word *nadi* refers to something that is flowing or to a hollow stalk or tube. In TCM, we use the word *meridian*, which comes from the term *jing luo*, meaning something that travels through or something that connects like a thread in a fabric. Like intricate threads of energy, these pathways join all body parts: they move and circulate vitality and nutrition; transmit information; and link every cell, organ, and Vital Substance. The ancient text the *Huang Di Nei Jing* (*The Inner Canon of the Yellow Emperor*), often referred to as the *Nei Jing*, points out how significant they are: "It is simply impossible that there is a place not passed through by the qi. This is like the flow of water, like the movement of sun and moon—they will never stop."[6]

Often, the twelve primary and two central meridians are emphasized when discussing the subtle body of TCM. Those are the meridians I use most frequently in my acupuncture practice. Each of the primary meridians has a specific relationship with an organ system. Consequently, when an internal organ is healthy, plenty of Qi will be circulating within its corresponding meridian and vice versa—a healthy meridian will have a positive, nourishing effect on its associated organ. However, it's also important to remember that a problem within a meridian can be a local issue in the channel itself and is not always related to its associated organ. For example, if I fall and sustain a muscle or bone injury along a meridian, it generally won't correlate with an internal organ imbalance. Instead, the stagnation will be local along whichever meridian lies in the area.

Beyond the primary pathways, many other meridians and internal tributaries comprise the complete latticelike network of your subtle body. Some channels diverge off the main meridians; there are tiny "minute" and "connecting" channels, and even "extraordinary" channels, that absorb excess Qi and Blood. Cutaneous regions support the surface of the body; we affect those when we use topical methods like massage or cupping.

We also have meridians called Sinew channels. These channels run along similar pathways to the primary meridians that we use with acupuncture and associate with the organs. They do not directly penetrate our organs but can reflect an imbalance in a primary meridian. Like the primary meridians, the Sinew channels are symmetrical and run on both sides of the body. Sinew channels are closely related to muscles and tendons, ligaments, and sensitive trigger points (*ashi* points). Unlike the primary meridians, which flow in a continual circuit, Sinew channels originate at the hands or feet and move inward. They also have a broader pathway, making them easier to locate, and they affect a larger area than the specific meridians used for acupuncture.

I find the Sinew channels especially relevant for bodyworkers, yogis, and movers because they directly relate to our connective tissue and fascia. Like a mycelial network or delicate spiderweb, the three-dimensional net of collagen-rich connective tissue we call fascia communicates and transmits information, nutrients, and vibrations similar to our energetic meridians. It also responds to movement. Connective tissue is what gives the living body uninterrupted and responsive integration from head to toe like the functions of the subtle body.

If we're sedentary, under stress, have poor posture, have experienced a physical trauma to our body, have lots of repetitive strain, or hold emotional states in our body, our fascia can tighten, thicken, and lose flexibility. When the fluid matrix of fascia dehydrates and locks up, our Qi and Blood get stuck and can't flow. Without flow, imbalance results. Like the layers of fascia in the body, meridians are constantly in the process of changing and reforming. Sinew channels are also said to express and contribute to the formation of our feelings. When we communicate emotions outwardly, we impact the Yang Sinew channels; when we suppress feelings, we influence the Yin Sinew channels.[7] This highlights how the energetic system influences and is affected by many layers of our being simultaneously.

When enough Qi moves freely through all our meridians, we feel great—we have very little pain, our emotions flow easily, and we are resilient when we encounter struggles. On the flip side, when Qi in the channel system is blocked or lacking somehow, we may feel stuck, depleted, or sensitive. Vibrant health depends on enough Qi moving through all the pathways of the subtle system in a smooth and harmonious flow. In TCM and Ayurveda, we affect our subtle channels (and therefore our energy) with everything we do—or don't do. For instance, in yoga, each delicate or gross movement can potentially touch the whole integrated network. However, we can also utilize many other intentional practices to affect this luminous web directly, which we'll explore next.

You'll find brief descriptions of the Sinew channels and main meridians for each organ and element in Part Two. For more information on the meridians, please visit wisdomofthebodybook.com.

WORKING WITH QI

Because Qi imbues our entire body-mind with life-giving energy, everything we do, think, and feel affects it. The foods we eat, the sleep we get, the way we move, where we live, the thoughts we think, the feelings we have, and the relationships we build all influence whether our energy is robust or deficient and whether it flows smoothly or erratically.

When we begin to work skillfully with our Qi through intentional practice, we become active participants in our own health and vitality. Regular use of methods that help us to harmonize and heal the flow of Qi in our bodies and minds has some specific benefits. First, working with our Qi serves our physical health. When we're used to checking in with our whole-body system, we're more likely to pick up on differences and changes early on, giving us the opportunity to alter our habits or lifestyle to address whatever is occurring. It also supports the body's natural intelligence—when we're energetically well, the physical body has an easier time adjusting and realigning with a state of balance. Next, by working with our subtle systems, we affect other interrelated spheres of our experience, including the mind, emotions, and spirit. When the subtle body system operates at a cleaner, more harmonious level, the mental sphere and spirit are calmer, less reactive, and more focused on the good of all. We'll explore these qualities in several ways throughout the book.

Here are a few main ways to affect your Qi; we'll explore direct practice in depth in Part Two.

NUTRITION AND HERBAL MEDICINES. Using food and herbs as medicine dates back thousands of years, and today, if you meet with a Chinese medicine practitioner like me, they will likely tell you which foods you should and should not eat and recommend herbal medicines that will treat your condition. Every meal is a chance to nourish and balance your energy based on your unique constitution and other factors like the season and your time of life. Luckily for us, early Ayurvedic and Chinese physicians codified a massive amount of information about the healing power of food and herbal medicines. For instance, every food has its own taste, thermal properties, affinity to specific organ systems, energetic direction, actions, and indications. Each of these qualities influences how it will affect our energy and condition. Understanding these energetic properties allows us to determine which foods suit our distinct needs. You'll find suggestions for every season and element in Part Two and specific recommendations around digestive health in Chapter 11. I recommend consulting a qualified herbalist if you wish to use herbal medicines.

MOVEMENT. Exercise of all kinds moves your Qi and blood, cleanses your organs, and keeps your muscles and bones healthy and strong. Like all suggestions from holistic medicine, finding your sweet spot is key. Too much exercise will deplete your body's energy, while not enough leaves you stagnant. Just the right amount is invigorating, nourishing, and mood-enhancing.

Holistic practices like yoga, somatic movement, Tai Ji, and Qi Gong are invaluable methods to encourage restoration and the distribution of Qi throughout your body. These wise systems use movements and postures to keep your tissues strong and adaptable and entice Qi into specific structures and organs. Practices in these traditions are designed to elicit your body's natural healing response and both stimulate and rejuvenate your deeper energetic structures, like your subtle body meridians. When you lengthen, twist, pump, pressurize, and decompress your body, you awaken the meridians and promote Qi and blood flow, which results in more vitality.

Lastly, these practices encourage mindful awareness, further enhancing and revitalizing Qi, which we'll explore later in this section.

ACUPUNCTURE AND ACUPRESSURE. The ancient physicians and sages identified specific places in the body where Qi accumulates or is more easily accessible. During acupuncture, we place fine, sterile pins just under the skin to work with the body's Qi and elicit a healing response. There are hundreds, if not thousands, of acupoints in the Chinese system; in acupuncture, we tend to focus mainly on the primary points, which total around 365. Acupuncturists must complete many years of rigorous, full-time academic study and professional board examinations to become licensed to practice.

You can use the same points in the body with acupressure. In acupressure, we stimulate these areas using massage, finger pressure, attention, intention, and even movement. With acupressure, we can balance, build, adjust, or sedate energy in much the same way as with acupuncture, albeit in a subtler way, depending on the imbalance that presents itself. It's interesting to note that many healing arts employ a similar concept of therapeutic points, including *marma* in Ayurveda. The functions and actions of each point can be complex, especially when using two or more points together, but there are still many ways to use the power of these points in your everyday life. We'll explore this more in Part Two.

Both TCM and Ayurveda use many other methods that rely on therapeutic touch. Here are a few from TCM: *tui na* (literally, "push and grasp") uses kneading, pressing, and rubbing to create relaxation and move Qi and Blood; *gua sha*, or "scraping," involves rubbing the skin with an implement that has smooth edges to create greater circulation; cupping uses a vessel to create a vacuum on the body, stimulating circulation and drawing out latent toxins; and moxibustion entails burning mugwort (*ai ye*) on or near specific areas of the body to warm and move Qi.

SENSE ORGAN CARE. Our senses act as bridges or portals between the external world of form and the inner world of the mind, feelings, and subtle energy. In TCM, each of our senses relates to an internal organ and elemental energy from the Five Elements, which we'll look at in the next chapter. In Ayurveda, misuse of the senses (*artha samyoga*) is one of three primary causes of disease. When our senses are under- or over-used, they cause agitation and interrupt our homeostasis. For instance, if we are in a state of constant stimulation and don't have a good balance between quiet time and the outward movement of attention through our senses, we will become drained. Working with the senses through various yoga and meditation techniques and regular self-care methods that nourish these organs of perception helps us regain balance. In Part Two, you'll find a healing practice for each sense organ that goes along with each of the Five Elements.

BREATHWORK. Deliberately engaging our breath (called *pranayama* in yoga) can profoundly alter and reinforce the strength and circulation of our Qi. By joining our attention with our breath, we automatically open ourselves to a world of possibility that includes revitalized tissues, sustained energy, and clarity of mind. Today, we have wisdom from the ancients regarding these practices, as well as many Western medical studies that further prove the positive physical and psychological impact of manipulating the breath for specific aims.

Many people have disordered breathing patterns that directly influence how vital they feel. Encouraging smooth and unrestricted breathing is the first step. This book offers many methods to tap into the various realms of your being; however, simple breath awareness is one you can continually revisit, no matter what other practices you're using. Working with specific breathing techniques can help you consciously engage your breath for deeper effects, which we'll explore more in later chapters.

MEDITATION. This final technique is the subtlest and perhaps the most profound. We can affect our Qi with our attention and intention using meditation, visualization, and inquiry practices. Like exercising the body, ancient Daoist and Indian yogis found that when they clarified or guided their minds, they could directly influence states of wellness and disease. I like to say that meditation is radical and revolutionary. In this fast-paced world that is so quick to distract us, meditation helps us rest in openness and be aware of and available for all experiences, whether terrifying, triumphant, or somewhere in between. A practice that teaches how to quiet the mind and be present is truly "countercultural"—and especially relevant today.

We also live in a culture that likes to hold on! Mindfulness is a practice that offers transformation through slowing the pace of reactivity and letting go. If your mental state is chaotic and your thoughts unruly, your out-of-control mind will drain your vital energy, distract you, and cause illness. In contrast, steadiness and spaciousness of mind help your energy and emotions flow smoothly and freely, supporting you in deeper energetic and spiritual healing.

The art and science of settling your mind and moderating your thoughts and emotions are not about trying to stop thinking and feeling. Instead, these are about understanding the nature of your mind by paying attention; gently controlling or transforming thoughts and emotions that cloud your clarity; and actively developing skillful states like kindness, tranquility, equanimity, compassion, and generosity. Developing mindful awareness also helps you be present enough to notice and parse out the internal messages from your body, mind, and spirit, thus better understanding energetic principles and your particularities.

Lastly, cultivating the mind can help you come to *know* your mind in a deeper way, to loosen the grip of harmful mind states and find more freedom, contentment, and joy. When you focus on the nature of consciousness or awareness itself, wisdom arises naturally. It is this wisdom that creates a kind of spaciousness and peace where inner healing happens more easily.

There are myriad practices that fit into the category of meditation, many of which we'll cover throughout this book. Some practices aim for relaxation, while others focus on building energy or insight. Generally speaking, beginning practices usually constellate around calming the mind and dwelling in the present moment. Regardless of their focus, these methods nourish our deepest life forces, keeping us well.

When preparing to meditate, you'll want to find a position of relative ease, usually with your spine upright, to create relaxation and alertness and help keep your energy channels flowing. This is especially important for the central channels, the *Sushumna* in the yoga system and the *Du* (Governing) and *Ren* (Conception) meridians in the Chinese system. Aim to have both *sthira* (steadiness) and *sukha* (ease) in your posture. Remember, there's nothing special about sitting cross-legged! It's more important to find a stable and comfortable place. Ideally, your meditation posture should encourage alignment of the skull, pelvis, and natural curves of the spine, along with a softening and widening of the respiratory diaphragm for easier breathing. I also suggest using a timer and keeping a shawl or light blanket handy to stay warm while practicing.

There are four traditional meditation postures: sitting, lying down, standing, and walking. I recommend you try all these postures, especially if you're new to practice or you've become accustomed to a specific one. Walking and standing meditation are particularly helpful if you experience pain while seated. Lying down is useful if you're unwell or fatigued. Whichever position you choose, adjust your posture if you begin experiencing a lot of discomfort; sometimes we can work with pain in our practice, but as a general rule, it's best to find a relatively manageable position. That way, we can focus on the internal practices of breath and body awareness rather than simply enduring and counting down the minutes.

Sitting is a fantastic meditation posture because it provides a solid base of support in the lower body while allowing your head, neck, and spine to align, which in turn supports a calm nervous system. Feel free to experiment with seated variations until you find something comfortable. To sit, ensure your hips are higher than your knees and you have a forward tilt in your pelvis. A cushion or blanket under your sitting bones can help you achieve this. If you sit cross-legged and your knees float away from the floor, you can place supports under them, but first check that your pelvis is tilted forward. If your lower back is rounding and your pelvis is tilted back, place more height under your sitting bones; if that doesn't work, try a different position. Try sitting on a soft surface and high enough that you can place the sides of your shins on the floor, with one foot in front of the other. Be sure your feet are not pressing against your legs as, over time, this will cause numbness in your legs and feet. You can also use cushions under your hands and arms for shoulder or neck tension.

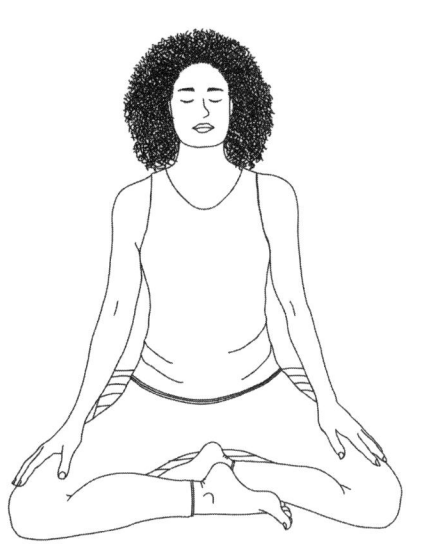

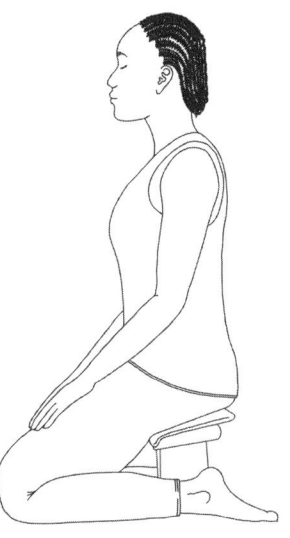

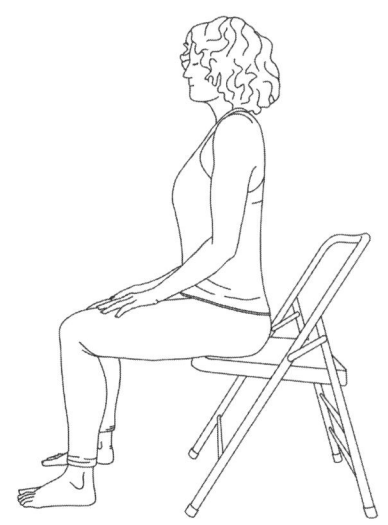

A meditation bench is another seated option to try—many medita-tors find a bench relieves a tight or sore lower back and cranky knees and hips. Or opt to sit in a chair. Always sit on the edge, away from the back, with your spine long and your pelvis tipped forward. Place both feet on the floor, and be sure your thigh bones are in a straight or des-cending line from your hips to your knees. Place a cushion under your hips or feet if they're not aligned.

For additional meditation tutorials, visit jenniferraye.com and the book's website at wisdomofthebodybook.com.

As you can see, Qi is a powerful life force that imbues absolutely every-thing with inherent energy. In our bodies, it both animates—and is the basis of—all structure in our tissues. This vital energy circulates through energetic pathways and expresses itself in our organs and bodily sub-stances. While it can go out of balance in a variety of ways, there are also many methods we can use to support, cultivate, and protect it. In the next chapter, we'll dive deeper into TCM theory to understand how to identify when we're out of balance, how we got there, and what to do about it.

TWO

HEALING WITH
EARTH-BASED MEDICINE

When those who are knowledgeable nourish their life, the following is for sure: They act in accordance with the four seasons
and adapt themselves to cold and summer heat. They harmonize
joy and anger, and they maintain calmness in their home. They
are moderate in regard to [making use of] their yin and yang [qi]
and they seek to find a balance between hard and soft. This way
they keep the evil away from them. They achieve longevity, and
their vision lasts long.[8]

—HUANG DI NEI JING

As we journey deeper into our body and mind, it will help to take a step
back first and understand some overarching concepts we'll use to guide
our path. In both Daoism and Sankhya, everything emerges out of the
limitless. In Daoism, we call this the Dao, or the Way. In Sankhya, this
is Brahma, an expression of an ultimate or supreme all-encompassing
reality.

As mentioned in the introduction, the Dao refers to a path or route.
This is no ordinary path, as this path can be internal—it guides us toward our true nature and the true nature of all things. Sometimes we
arrive on the path disheveled or lost. At other times we go out searching
for it or inadvertently stumble upon it. Fortunately for us, the inner path
has been traversed by the many seekers who came before us. These

voyagers left signposts, detailed instructions, and encrypted messages along the way to guide our journey home, like the intricate maps of the subtle body we explored in the last chapter. Their directions not only apply to our bodies, they also refer to the patterns of our whole universe. The travelers who walked this way before us understood that the fundamental rules governing all things outside us can also be essential allies and guides for our journey within.

YIN AND YANG

As for water and fire, they are the signs of yin and yang. As for yin and yang, they are the beginning of the myriad beings.[9]
—HUANG DI NEI JING

In Daoism and TCM, all things are born from the infinite source of the Dao. The foundational qualities of Yin and Yang arise out of this formless void and create our manifest world. In yoga, this is similar to *Brahmana* and *Langhana*—nourishing and activating qualities and lightening and calming qualities, respectively. Water and fire, sunset and sunrise, and every exhalation and inhalation are Yin and Yang at play. Yin and Yang symbolize a dynamic duality and beautifully represent how opposite forces are complementary and interdependent in our natural world. Although these two forces appear distinct, they are constantly emerging and transforming in concert with one another. They are divisible yet inseparable.

Think of the Yin-Yang symbol. The dark side of the symbol (Yin) represents reality's introverted and dense aspect—coldness, darkness, yielding, and slowness. Its Chinese character is the shady or north side of a mountain. The light side of the symbol (Yang) represents the sunny or south side. Its energies are more immaterial; extroverted; and associated with more activity, heat, light, and movement. Nothing can ever be completely Yin or Yang. The light side still contains a tiny seed of Yin (the dark dot), and the dark side still contains a tiny seed of Yang (the light dot).

The terms *Yin* and *Yang* are relative, meaning we can only define these energies in comparison to each other. For example, when Daoists use Yin and Yang to describe our cosmos, the heavens are Yang, and the earth is Yin. However, if we're only speaking of earth, then whatever is denser or more interior is Yin, while what is active or dynamic is Yang. You can see this in our bodies too. The top half of the body is more Yang, while the bottom half is more Yin. But if we only speak of the bottom of the body—say, the legs—then the outer leg is more Yang, and the inner leg is more Yin.

Because of their dynamic nature, you can also think of Yin and Yang as phases of a cyclical movement that fluidly transform into one another. Sometimes one will be more dominant because of the continually shifting nature of time. Just as day turns to night, activity requires rest, youth progresses to old age, and the seasons follow a pattern of heat and cold and light and dark, Yin and Yang are in a vital state of constant change. They may not transform naturally or at a good time, but it will inevitably happen. Let's say you have a high fever (Yang). Eventually, it will transform into shock, and your body will become cold (Yin). Essentially, the natural order of things is biased toward balance, so extremes cause transformation and a return to homeostasis.

Disharmony results when the balance of Yin and Yang is interrupted or thrown out of whack. Because Yin and Yang are so closely interdependent and intertwined, when one is weak, the other will increase. If it's a hot summer, for example, and you're under a lot of stress and eating a lot of energetically hot foods, you may cause a buildup of hot Yang qualities and lack the cooling, moistening Yin qualities your body needs. As a result, you may feel hot or agitated; be excessively thirsty; or have heartburn, a dry red rash, or constipation. However, Yang can also provide the right amount of warmth and energy. If it's winter and you've been sedentary and eating a lot of iced and cold foods, Yin-like qualities will increase because you lack Yang's warmth. In that case, you may be cold and pale and experience weak digestion, water retention, low libido, fatigue, or slowness in movement.

Keeping in mind that we need both Yin and Yang and that they balance and temper each other, we can look to our yoga and lifestyle practices to emphasize one quality more than the other. In yoga, we balance active and passive qualities by regulating solar and lunar energies in our bodies and minds. Passive and slow movements are more lunar or Yin, while fast and dynamic movements are more solar or Yang. As you deepen your practice of mindful awareness with regular yoga and meditation and by engaging the methods in this book, you'll begin to recognize qualities in your body-mind or environment as having more of one than the other.

Equipped with this information, you can aim to balance your Yin-Yang energies by doing a practice that strengthens the opposite. You may have a very busy, fiery, and active life. In that case, working with more Yin-style practices—being quieter, holding postures longer, or working with relaxation practices—will create balance. Even so, you may still want to include some Yang aspects in your Yin-style practice—adding methods that clarify the mind or breathwork that is more heating—to represent the seed of Yang within Yin. If you lean toward being more Yin—say, you work at a desk job and are relatively introverted—you may want to create balance with a more vigorous heating practice but still include some meditation at the end or beginning of your practice for that seed of Yin.

You can also work with Yin and Yang using seasonal practices. For instance, spring is a time of "Yang within Yin," or Yang rising, meaning energy is transitioning from the Yin season (winter) to the Yang season (summer). To attune to this energy, you might bring in more active practices (Yang) to help awaken and enliven your energy. Or perhaps it's autumn; in that case, you're in the "Yin within Yang" season, or Yin rising, transitioning from summer to winter. You may want to bring in more restorative practices to help you slow down and rest more.

Looking at the preceding examples, you may notice at some point that increasing the same energy that is present becomes too much. As summer approaches, the heating practices you used in spring might be too active; instead, to create balance, you'll want to use cooling, Yin-type practices that help ground and settle your energy as temperatures and activities outside increase. The same goes for your autumn practices. If you start to feel too sluggish as winter approaches and deepens, you'll need to reduce the slower, Yin-style practices that worked so well in autumn in favor of something more dynamic.

This isn't to say that you can never follow your preferred inclinations (doing a heating practice in summer or a cooling one in winter, for example), but if that's all you ever do, balance and good health will be more difficult to achieve. Ultimately, when there's an imbalance of Yin and Yang energies, there's the potential for disease, and finding our perfect homeostasis at any given time creates optimal health.

THE RHYTHM OF NATURE

The ancient Daoists knew that the movements of the natural world were no different than the shifting landscape of our bodies, minds, and spirits, so through observation of natural phenomena, they outlined the system of the *Wu Xing*, or Five Elements. *Wu* means "five," and *Xing* means "process, movement, phase, or behavior." It's interesting to note that many traditional medical systems have categories of elements. Greek philosophers, Native American healers, and Ayurvedic practitioners all use a system of elements to describe dynamic qualities in nature. In Ayurveda and yoga, the elements are Space, Air, Fire, Water, and Earth; in TCM, they are Wood, Fire, Earth, Metal, and Water.

The details of the most ancient shamanic underpinnings of the Five Elements have been lost to antiquity; however, the TCM text the *Nei Jing* (which includes the *Su Wen* and the *Ling Shu*) and the *Vedas*—a collection of ancient texts that form the foundation of Ayurveda and yoga, representing India's scholarship and wisdom—outline the elements and how we can relate to them skillfully.

In TCM, the Five Elements highlight the concept that energy slowly changes through phases, qualities, movements, or patterns—just like Yin and Yang. It gives us another mythical map of the divine pattern of things. Rather than fixed points, the Five Elements symbolize the cycle of life. Wood is a time for growth and expansion, similar to spring. Fire represents heat and maximum function and is an upward movement, like summer. Earth is a time of balance and nourishment, representing a center point or transitionary period between each season. Metal is a declining or decaying state and a time of contraction, like autumn. Water is a time of rest; it represents the darkness and downward movement that is akin to winter.

These five phases are usually portrayed in a circle, illustrating the progression of all life, with each element proceeding from the last. A circle is enduring; it suggests the cyclical nature of time and energy. When considering the circle, I think of the complex and multifaceted Tibetan mandalas that illustrate our universe and inner terrain. The circle represents the dynamic display of energy in nature and all things within a timeless container of continuity.

Just like nature cycles through the Five Elements, so do we. We begin in the dark and watery realm of the womb, just like a seed buried deep beneath the earth. Eventually, that seed sprouts and grows toward the light as we do throughout our adult life, perhaps encountering obstacles that hinder our growth or encourage adaptability. Then we reach full blossoming and expression and heightened activity, which quickly transforms into maturation and nourishment in the form of the fruits of life. Soon our leaves drop, and letting go takes over as we return to the earth to feed the soil and cycle all over again.

In TCM, the generation cycle shows the elements in balance: Wood feeds Fire, Fire regenerates Earth, Earth creates Metal, Metal collects Water, and Water grows Wood. Each element supports and contributes to the next phase. For example, Wood may not get enough energy if Water is weak. The control or destruction cycle is the other main cycle. It follows the route of a five-pointed star inside the circle. If that relationship is healthy, we call it a control cycle because everything stays in balance, but if there's too much control, it becomes a destruction cycle. For instance, in my clinical practice, I often see patients who experience an excess of the Wood element (stress, headaches, anger). With time, excess Wood eventually overcontrols Earth through the destruction cycle (refer to the inner arrows in the diagram on page 37), leading to Earth element problems like weakened digestion. To maintain health and vitality in the natural world and our bodies and minds, we need a balance of these energies. The *Dao De Jing* says it this way: "For all things, there is a time for going ahead, and a time for following behind;

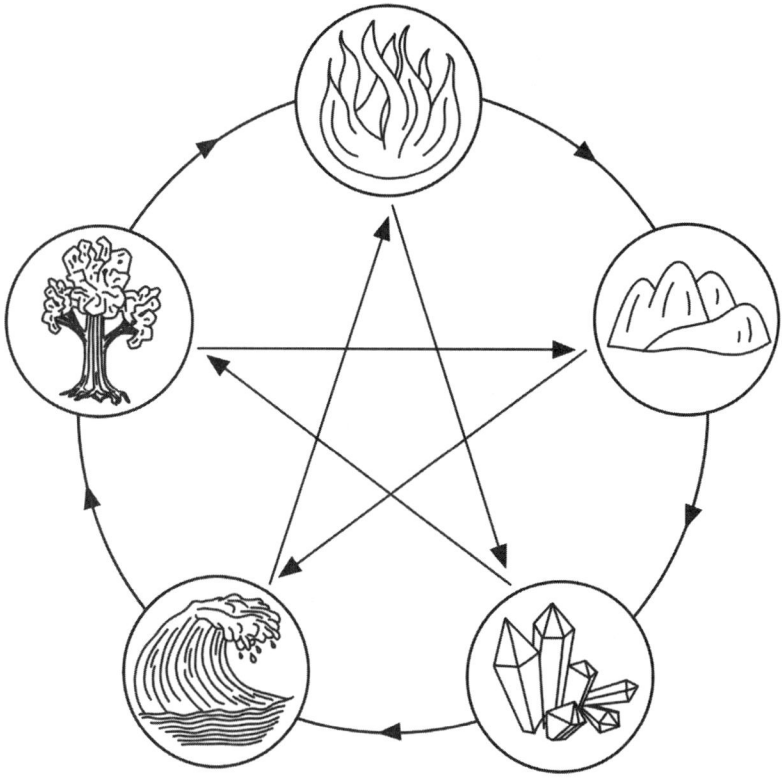

A time for slow-breathing and a time for fast-breathing; A time to grow in strength and a time to decay."[10]

It is important to understand that each element has a particular resonance or frequency, which gives it specific characteristics. You can think of each of the Five Elements or phases as having their own sound or hum, and everything in the universe will or will not resonate with this note. This is what determines how we associate specific elements with aspects of nature and even distinct parts of our bodies and minds. In Part Two, we'll deeply explore how each element has a related season, movement, color, body tissue, organ system, set of meridians, emotion, and spiritual characteristics. These connections happen because all of these features have similar energies or, you could say, *vibrate* at the same rate. When we learn to adapt our bodies and minds to the cycle of these great archetypes, we align with the cycles of nature, creating a harmonious sound that equals vibrant health.

ENERGETICS OF IMBALANCE

There are only a few main causes underlying all imbalances, according to TCM and Ayurveda. In Ayurveda and yoga, our constitutional energy gives us our basic design, then we look to imbalances related to three main factors as the causes of disease. They are time (*kala*), such as the seasons or aging; the misuse of our intellect (*prajnaparadha*), for instance when our actions or choices don't take into account the wisdom of our body; and the over- or underuse of our senses (*artha samyoga*), such as too much or too little stimulation for our eyes or ears. I mentioned the last one in Chapter 1 when we covered some practices to support healthy Qi. In TCM, the main drivers of disharmony are divided into three categories: external conditions, like infectious diseases; internal causes, such as those that develop as a result of disordered mental or emotional states; and a third category that encompasses other considerations, for instance constitution and lifestyle choices like diet, activity levels, overwork, excess sexual behavior, and sleep habits as well as factors like parasites and wrong medical treatment. If you pay attention to these causes, you'll be well on your way to treating and preventing many imbalances. While it's beyond the scope of this book to parse out every detail of how these two systems are alike and different, let's look at a few main factors that contribute to imbalance that these systems so elegantly identify.

Constitution

Your constitution is a special gift. Because we are an essential part of nature and the flow of time, we are each given specific attributes and energy levels to fulfill our distinct destinies. Your personality and body may change as you move through life, but your underlying constitutional framework remains pretty much the same. The health of your ancestors is what primarily influences this set of characteristics, especially the health of your parents and of your mother during pregnancy.

In Ayurveda, your constitution comprises a unique set of elemental energies we call your *prakriti*. In TCM, we also look to the elements to determine which is most prominent. This is why these systems don't have uniform suggestions that apply to everyone. We each have a unique makeup of elements; therefore, the energetic qualities we exhibit will be different.

In TCM, you likely have a robust constitution if you have consistently good energy and spirits and healthy physical features like firm muscles and lustrous skin. Perhaps you know someone blessed with an exceptionally sturdy makeup. This person usually doesn't encounter any significant health issues during childhood and remains resilient and well throughout life without much effort. When a person with a strong constitution encounters challenges, they typically bounce back fairly quickly and without long-term consequences. People with constitutional weakness struggle more to maintain health—they may have developmental problems as children and are more likely to bear chronic or inherited illnesses.

While discovering your constitution is not covered in this book, a few techniques may be helpful to start the process. Constitutional quizzes are out there; however, I find they're not always very accurate because constitutional analysis can be nuanced. As you explore all the concepts in this book, especially the Five Elements in Part Two, pay special attention to how they apply to your proclivities and aversions. Do you prefer winter or summer? Is there a specific climate in which your body and mind seem to thrive? What about how you were throughout childhood? What kinds of leanings did you have then? Were you a quiet kid, or did you prefer lots of socializing and activity? What kind of imbalances do you tend to get? Are they hot or cold, dry or damp? We'll explore some of these factors and more throughout our investigation. Lastly, I often recommend that patients and students start a journal to track their physical and mental health. Take note of things like sleep changes, digestion, and predominant moods. You may discover specific patterns you wouldn't have seen otherwise.

The unique grouping of capacities and challenges we are born with is out of our control. Still, we can positively affect our constitutional traits and nurture good health using foods, herbal medicines, lifestyle choices, and practices. We'll keep exploring all of that in upcoming chapters.

Subtle Qualities

One way we can become imbalanced, according to these systems, is not having enough, or having too much, of certain qualities. For instance, the Five Elements in Ayurveda and TCM each have certain characteristics. If these attributes are excessive or deficient, we may experience imbalance. In Ayurveda, we identify specific qualities (*gunas*) like dryness, roughness, mobility, or cold that go along with specific elements and states of health and disease—physically, mentally, and even spiritually. For example, Fire has the quality of heat; it contributes to everything from breaking down food during digestion to driving your ambition to supporting the clarity of your mind. This is similar in TCM. Each of the Five Elements we looked at earlier has specific resonances or qualities.

We associate energetic characteristics or resonances with certain elements, and they can arise at particular times in our lives, at certain times of day, or during specific seasons. For example, you might notice dryness increasing in your body as you enter your senior years. In TCM, we describe this as a Yin, Blood, or Body Fluid depletion. In Ayurveda, there is an increase in Space and Air elements. Either way, the increasing characteristic is dryness, leading to dry hair, nails, and skin, as well as weaker bones and so on.

In TCM, we also use the language of the pathogens to describe certain energetic influences. They are Wind, Cold, Heat, Dampness, Dryness, and Summer Heat. Each pathogen relates to an element in the Five Element model, a season, and an internal organ, as you'll see when we get to Part Two. In TCM, all pathogens except Summer Heat can arise either inside the body or from our external environment. They can occur separately or in combination with each other. In Chinese medicine, pathogens both name an imbalance and describe its cause; for example, a red rash is a Heat condition due to the buildup of the pathogen Heat. Medical texts also name Phlegm and Blood stasis as pathogens that are not directly related to the Five Elements and seasons and will not be covered here.

In TCM, if a pathogen occurs externally, it's usually identifiable by its rapid onset and its symptoms affecting the nose, mouth, throat, lungs, or skin, such as fever, chills, aches, sore throat, rashes, sneezing and sweating. This includes Western medicine's understanding of bacteria and viruses in the environment, which affect Qi related to immunity that circulates near the surface of your body (Wei Qi). External pathogens are only a problem if the body cannot protect itself. Depending on the strength of your body's defense, you'll either get sick or fight off the influence. However, even healthy people can be affected if a pathogen attack is strong enough. For instance, think of sunstroke on a scorching day or coming down with a chill when you didn't adequately cover your neck during a windy hike. Pathogens can even affect the body in artificial environments. I once had a patient who worked in a refrigerated environment who had health issues due to long-term exposure to the Cold pathogen.

Internal pathogens are usually more chronic or longer term and are typically caused by poor lifestyle choices leading to an imbalance in your energetic organs, strength, and vitality over time. Let's briefly look at the pathogens outlined in TCM as they relate to the Five Elements and how they affect us.

WIND. Think of how Wind in the natural world arouses movement. It is a Yang energy that is light, dry, airy, erratic, and rapid. Just as the wind sweeps leaves off the forest floor, Wind in the body causes turbulent, irregular movement and things to appear and disappear quickly. External Wind invasion can lead to seasonal allergies and common colds; if left unchecked, it can become lodged in your body, developing into lung congestion and longer-term fatigue. Wind can also develop internally with irregular and chaotic symptoms, such as twitching, tremors, numbness, disturbed vision, flatulence, and dizziness. In this case, we typically look to the Liver and the Wood element, which are responsible for the smooth flow of Qi.

COLD. Cold is a Yin energy that indicates a lack of warmth or Yang. Just as cold causes water to turn to ice, the Cold pathogen in your body slows your systems and contracts tissues. With Cold, whether it begins externally or internally, you may feel chilled, have poor circulation, look pale, experience pain relieved by warmth, exhibit a lack of thirst, and move slowly and sluggishly. In my clinical practice, I often see women who experience infertility or severe menstrual cramps from Cold. Often, we cause imbalance through overexposure to a cold, damp environment and a poor diet. If the Cold is internal, it may stem from an energetic weakness in your Water element and energetic Kidneys leading to exhaustion, sore knees, and lower back pain. Cold can also combine with digestive weakness and lead to insufficient digestive capacity and loose stools. In this case, we look to the energetic Spleen and the Earth element.

HEAT. The nature of Heat is Yang; it is warming and activating. Excess heat in our environment causes the earth to dry and crack. Heat in the body can cause Body Fluids to dry, leading to inflammation, dry stools, thirst, and scanty urination. Other symptoms may include infection; a feeling of heat; red skin issues; a strong appetite; and bleeding problems such as excessive menstruation or, in extreme cases, hemorrhage. Too much Heat can point to the Fire element, but it can also implicate the Wood element if stagnant Qi is causing the Heat (the Wood element is responsible for smooth flow). If Heat is due to an internal Yin deficiency, you'll experience night sweats; hot palms, chest, and feet; and anxiety or insomnia. In this case, we often look to the Water element. Heat can also affect your mind, leading to restlessness, mania, and even spiritual disturbance. Summer Heat is another pathogen that is a more pronounced case of Heat. It only manifests externally.

DAMPNESS. Dampness is a sticky, heavy, wet, and downward-moving Yin energy that accumulates. External Dampness from your environment will cause your symptoms to worsen in cold, wet climates. For example, joint pain that acts up during humid or damp weather. Internal Dampness, however, is most often connected to Qi deficiency—especially Earth element and Spleen Qi deficiency. Chapter 11 notes that when our Spleen Qi is not strong enough, our digestive fire can't properly digest food and drink, leading to Dampness. When Dampness builds up in your body-mind, it feels like a heavy fog. Rather than eliminating stagnant fluids, your body holds on to them and becomes dull and dense. Symptoms of internal Dampness include poor digestion; a feeling of heaviness; excessive worry or thinking; edema; weight gain; a thick, greasy coating on the tongue; poor appetite; and loose stools.

DRYNESS. Dryness is a pathogen characterized by a lack of fluid. Symptoms include dry nostrils, tongue, and lips; rough or flaky skin; dry stools; and constipation. Dry air in the environment, such as a long day in an air-conditioned office or outside on a ski hill, can quickly dry the body out, leading to dehydration and dry sinuses. For this, we usually balance the Metal element and Lungs. Long-term Dryness can also indicate deficient Blood, Body Fluids, and Yin. Sometimes, internal Dryness is due to energetic Kidney depletion.

Mind and Emotions

In Ayurveda and yoga, karma is central to understanding how imbalance and disease arise. The meaning of *karma* implies both action and reaction. Essentially, everything we do, say, and think has consequences—for good or bad. Each of our choices starts with an urge in the mind. When we're healthy, our desires reflect a balanced mind, which leads to better choices. When we're making decisions that are bad for us—even though a deeper part of us knows what would be healthy—we create the conditions for suffering, and it's considered an imbalance in the mind.

Emotions also play a central role in disease causation. In TCM, all illnesses have an emotional or psychological component. Did you know the term *emotion* comes from the Latin *emovere*, which means "to move outward" and the French *emouvoir*, meaning "to excite"?[11] Emotions are simply energy moving and can have positive and negative aspects. When emotions go on for too long, are extreme, are sudden, are held on to, or are not expressed, they can cause imbalance, disease, and illness. Conversely, when a person experiences persistent issues with a specific organ, they may feel an increase in its related emotions. Emotions also hold a very important key to developing our spiritual nature, according to the ancients. Each element has an associated higher spiritual virtue, and when we're unhealthy, these virtues degrade into their associated emotional expression.

TCM recognizes seven central emotional tones: anger, joy (over-excitement), rumination, sadness or grief, worry or anxiety, fear, and shock. Each is linked with an element and an organ: anger, related to the Liver and Wood element, rises upward; joy and shock relate to the Heart and Fire element and loosen or disperse our energy; worry and rumination pertain to the Spleen and Earth element and cause our energy to knot; grief or sadness, connected to the Lungs and Metal element, leads to a deflation or dissipation of energy; and fear, which we link to the Kidneys and Water element, causes our energy to sink or freeze. Essentially, mind states and emotions leave an energetic imprint on the body-mind and directly affect our actions, whether good or bad. We'll explore emotions and how to transform them in detail in Part Two.

A Note on Stress

Life will always have stressful times, so the key is finding a balance between too much and too little, learning ways to build your capacity to handle stress, and returning to a baseline of calm after stressful events. Our hardwired stress response should be short-lived, but the problem I encounter in my clinic is that it's no longer a temporary occurrence for many folks and persists well past the initial stressor. I probably don't have to tell you that many of us encounter too much chronic low-grade stress and overstimulation without much time to relax or discharge the effects of that stress. So, instead of protecting us, our stress response damages us and disrupts our natural biological rhythms. Whether worrying about the state of the world, job security, health, or relationship struggles, chronic long-term exposure to stressful circumstances lowers immunity; causes sleep, digestive, and endocrine troubles; and contributes to tissue degeneration.

Along with a healthy diet, moderate exercise, and cultivating healthy relationships, Chinese medicine teaches us to look to each of the individual elements and organ systems for guidance in healing this over-activated response. For instance, stress often causes Qi stagnation in the body-mind, which leads to Wood element symptoms like a tendency toward anger, headaches, or depression. With Wood element dominance, there is a higher likelihood of addiction. Stress that's connected to shock or trauma results in such Fire element symptoms as anxiety, insomnia, or heart palpitations. If your Fire element is dominant, you may tend to avoid your stress through escapism. In the extreme, Fire-type stress can manifest as mania or bipolar disorder. Digestive concerns or disordered eating when you're stressed are signs of Earth element imbalance. If your Earth is more dominant, you may have weight gain or loss, and you may react to stress by seeking comfort in unhealthy foods or relationships with unhealthy boundaries. When your Metal element is stressed, symptoms will generally appear as body pain, in the large intestine as constipation, in the lungs with breathing difficulties like panic attacks, or in the immune system with frequent colds and sinus infections. With Metal element dominance, you may become more rigid and fixated on work, doing things right, or "following the rules," or you may use spiritual practices to dissociate. Chronic overwhelm and exhaustion leading to burnout is an indication of Water element involvement. With Water element dominance, the tendency is to isolate, feel numb, or experience bouts of fatigue. Part Two will cover more on this topic.

Now that we've covered some foundational concepts and terminology, we can turn our attention to how these wise traditions determine what particular pattern we have. We'll also explore how we might apply all this insight to four interrelated spheres of our being—physical, energetic, mental, and spiritual.

THREE

THE INNER PATH

When a person's natural endowment is kept intact, the spirit is harmonious, the eyes clear, the ears acute, the nose keen, the mouth perceptive, and the 360 joints of the body move smoothly. Such a person is trusted without speaking, acts exactly as needed without devising schemes, and succeeds without planning ahead. His vital essence circulates through Heaven and Earth and his spirit covers the cosmos. Of material things, there are none he does not accept and none he does not encompass— in this he is like Heaven and Earth . . . Such a man may be said to keep his power intact.[12]

—THE ANNALS OF LÜ BUWEI

To reestablish or maintain our health, we first need to identify what, in TCM, we call a "pattern of disharmony." One of the profound insights holistic medicine offers us is that health and disease exist on a spectrum. Illness usually manifests over time in small increments (excluding unexpected acute injuries). Instead of a disease state arriving suddenly, seemingly out of nowhere, subtle signs arise in the body and mind as the imbalance happens piece by piece. For instance, many stress-related diseases or chronic health problems don't simply spring up overnight. Instead, they slowly become more apparent. If we identify and address the early signs, we can avoid full-blown illnesses that require severer interventions. This is a significant distinction that sets holistic systems apart from other forms of medicine, and it's at the core of how TCM and Ayurveda diagnose and treat energetic conditions before they become more difficult-to-handle diseases. In holistic medicine, we can work with patterns present at any time to create balance, even if we're relatively healthy.

For example, once you know how to look for signs of Qi stagnation in the body—such as an increased propensity to feel stuck or tense—you can circumvent more serious Qi stagnation conditions, like depression, by exercising (which moves stagnant Qi) as soon as you feel the early symptoms creeping in. Or you may have signs of Yang deficiency, like cold hands and feet. If you don't address it with practices that help build Yang, this minor symptom may progress into severer signs later in life, such as arthritis, which worsens with cold weather. As you can see, identifying the underlying imbalance allows you to change the pattern early so it doesn't progress along a spectrum from health to disease.

In the modern developed world, we're often encouraged to avoid pain or discomfort at all costs. We tend to mask our symptoms without looking into what caused them in the first place or what they are telling us about our state of health. While there may be times when we need a quick fix to get on with our day, if we ignore the underlying cause of our symptoms, our suffering will most likely return with louder and louder messages. Whereas Western medicine is often reductionist and emphasizes singular agents of disease, holistic systems understand the larger energetic language of the body-mind and catch trends early on, allowing us to shift our choices and offset whatever has become out of balance.

For instance, during a consultation with a patient, I gather a diverse set of data looking for broad trends rather than singular symptoms. By observing, inquiring, listening, smelling, and using palpation, I assess the overall internal landscape or "pattern" that my patient is exhibiting. I might listen to the tone or strength of their voice, assess their complexion, take their pulse, look at their tongue, and ask many seemingly unrelated questions. All this information helps me establish what pattern is present. Do they have too much Dampness? Or not enough Yin? How is their Kidney Qi? Is it deficient? What about their Liver Blood? Is it stagnant?

In TCM, one symptom can indicate vastly different patterns of imbalance, and we sometimes treat different diseases using the same method. For example, multiple patients might have a headache, but to treat each one, I need to differentiate the *kind* of headache they have. Is it due to Blood deficiency? Liver Qi stagnation? Wind, Cold, or Heat? Just some of the factors that will help me determine the specific pattern each patient has are things like their general constitution, how they sleep, the time of day they get a headache, where on their head they feel it, and what their digestion and/or menstruation is like. I could also have two patients who have entirely different complaints—let's say one has insomnia, while the other complains of fatigue. I might end up giving these two patients similar treatments or suggesting a similar herbal formula because, after examining and questioning them, I determine they both have the same pattern of imbalance underlying their condition, such as Blood deficiency. As you can see, Chinese medicine diagnosis is not as simple as naming a symptom. We need to understand the underlying pattern of imbalance before we can address it.

Once we've distinguished a specific pattern, we can correct it using practices and remedies that counteract the trend. Suppose you experience Cold symptoms that worsen in cold weather. In that case, eating more energetically warming foods during fall and winter will balance the effect of Cold in the environment. Everyone is unique, so TCM also tailors solutions and remedies to individuals depending on their tendencies and constitution. One person's joint pain may worsen with cold or damp weather, while another may have a history of gastric troubles and find that their joint pain flares up when they eat too much sugar. The first person will want to protect against Cold, while the other will focus on getting to the root of inflammation caused by insufficient digestive capacity.

This method allows us to adapt solutions as patterns in the body-mind change. After all, we humans are organisms that are constantly changing, and our always-shifting environment and choices directly influence how health and disease manifest in our body-mind. Our diet, sleep, exercise, age, genetics, environment, culture, and relationships all affect our state of equilibrium. Therefore, the remedies and medicine needed to maintain or reestablish balance should be adaptable and account for these factors. That same person with the winter joint pain might discover that, when they're overly active during hot summer months and enjoy a lot of hot, spicy food, they can't sleep and suffer from red, itchy eyes—both Heat signs. In that case, they will want to *reduce* heating activities and foods in the summer and continue to increase them in the winter.

Lastly, it's important to mention that healing or addressing imbalance at this level doesn't always mean our unpleasant symptoms will automatically disappear—especially when they are more extreme or have progressed. Sometimes, good health means learning to live with an illness in a well-balanced way. The key is that we start from the assumption of wholeness, that symptoms are simply clues that something is out of whack. Paying attention to patterns helps us focus on the root cause, supports our inherent wisdom and healing capacity, and creates the right environment for vital health to emerge naturally.

You, too, can understand yourself better and learn what might help you heal and what might be making you feel unwell by looking at collections of signs and symptoms. Your symptoms may have a Western medical diagnosis; however, when we look at them through the framework we'll explore throughout this book, you'll understand the nature of the condition and why the pattern is developing. From there, you can work with your practices, diet, lifestyle, or environment to create more balance and improve your health.

BODIES OF HEALING

Healing in the deepest and innermost way requires integration at all levels of being: physical, energetic, mental, and spiritual. Moreover, all ventures in life have outer and inner facets, or gross and subtle aspects. To skillfully bring holistic medicine into our lives, we must learn to meet our experience with care and determine what type or degree of health and healing we're ready and willing to work with. We each need to assess where on the continuum of integration we lie at a given moment. For instance, some of us require more or less nurturance on the physical plane of our bodies. Others are prepared to mine the depths of their psyches, while still others may find working with the imaginal realm of metaphor, myth, and dream helpful and illuminating.

This isn't to say that one aspect of your being is more important. In fact, quite the opposite. We all need inner and outer, subtle and gross practices, remedies, and technologies to stay well. Our needs are like the changing landscape of the seasons. They shift and transform like the phases of the moon or the tides of the great oceans. As wayfarers on the path, we must plot a course through the many twists and turns and strange and wonderful gifts we encounter along the way—be they delicate and elusive or tangible and substantial. The trick is to choose the right method at the appropriate time along the vast spectrum of options.

The holistic paradigms we've been exploring connect us with the true *spanda*, or "pulse" of life. They help us heal or attend to all the disordered, disintegrated, and shadow aspects of our being in the service of wholeness. They do this by attuning us to the deeper promptings, rhythms, and cycles of the body, mind, and heart as well as the natural world. In this way, they aid in energy cultivation and a deeper form of healing. Through the practices and techniques these systems offer, we can learn to open to the fleeting moments of our lives with awareness, patience, and care. This can assist us in integrating what is unacknowledged or difficult, and it can help us to see, feel, and respond to our inner and outer circumstances fully and skillfully.

For instance, at times your healing—and therefore your yoga practice—may emphasize more physical benefits. We all need movement and must engage our physicality to remain healthy and vital. In this case, you might use asanas, or postures, to build the musculoskeletal layer of your body for both stability and mobility. However, within the healing arts, the different realms of our being are not usually mutually exclusive. While you may choose to emphasize one focus on any particular day, your practices and therapeutic actions will still touch and affect the whole integrated network of your being. In fact, it's rare to find practices that simply focus on one domain of existence. For example, I may choose to do a physically demanding movement practice that challenges my body that also has a secondary effect of helping me feel more confident or emotionally/psychologically stronger.

In Chinese medicine, health is cultivated and maintained through practices called *yang sheng*, which means "to nourish/nurture life or vitality." These practices include developing the mind and emotions; regulating diet, sleep, and activity levels; caring for children, enjoying nature and art; having a healthy sex life; and managing specific times of life like pregnancy and old age. Ayurveda comes from the root word *ayur*, meaning "life," and translates as the "science of life." It also has a system of self-care rooted in principles that emphasize the importance of diet, sleep, moderating activity levels, working with the mind, and taking care of ourselves based on age and constitution. Both systems use diet; herbal medicine; therapeutic bodywork; and daily, seasonal, and life-stage rhythms to address the root causes of dis-ease, some of which we touched on earlier.

Next we'll cover the four main areas these wisdom traditions help us adjust, enhance, and support.

The Physical and Subtle Body

The therapeutic approaches in TCM and Ayurveda most definitely nourish life on the material plane, including your denser aspects— your muscles, bones, nerves, and physical organs. In yoga, the physical body is the *annamayakosha* (literally "food body"). We explored earlier how much of your physical body is set at birth with your constitution, like your propensity toward certain conditions, but you can also continue to influence it—often drastically—through the decisions you make and the lifestyle and mindset you have. Learning to be aware of and work with this gross aspect of your being can be very effective. Personally appropriate daily rhythms, movement, diet, and forms of bodywork can all go a long way to healing the physical body. Attending to this aspect of your being can begin with simply paying attention to a few breaths and checking in ("How am I feeling now?"). Once you're more connected to the present moment as lived and expressed in and through your body, you're more able to make adjustments based on your particular needs.

We've explored how our physical bodies also contain worlds within that are far beyond the muscles, tendons, and bones that make up our structure. The energetic sphere of your being that circulates Qi and animates your energetic organs and meridians is less tangible but no less important. In yoga we call this layer of being the *pranamayakosha* (breath and energy body). Ancient wisdom teachings recognize that we must also look to this more delicate aspect of our reality to remain healthy. Even though traditions vary in exactly how this subtle interior domain is mapped, explored, and worked with, many similarities remain. For instance, in both Chinese and Indian traditions, we access the subtle body using methods like movement, breathing techniques, meditation, and intentions. Our senses are often the doorway into this vast inner reality. Your subtle body lives in your physical body and strongly reflects your moods, emotions, and mental states. This energy body may be invisible, but you can still feel it. As you train in attending to the energetic layer of your being through the practices in this book, you will begin to sense it more deeply and develop a richer relationship with it.

The Mind and Emotions

There is also the mental realm of your multifaceted self, which includes your thoughts, memories, sense impressions, feelings, and emotions. In yoga, this is the *manomayakosha* (mental and emotional body). This layer is deeply interconnected and highly reliant on both your physicality and subtle body and vice versa. Your thoughts, feelings, and emotions can manifest in physical symptoms, and your mental health is impacted by how physically healthy you are. Ancient Daoists put a lot of focus on this realm and often emphasized the importance of regulating the mind for overall vitality, longevity, and well-being. The last chapter covered how, in TCM, our emotions are one of only a few central causes of disease. The ancients recognized that thought and emotion often agitate us and lead to physical manifestations and subtle body changes like Qi and Blood stagnation.

Daoist texts often describe our emotions as natural phenomena, like great winds that disturb our peace or scatter our Qi. However, they also emphasize that good health is not about having no emotion at all.

Rather, it is about not allowing emotion, thought, or mental disturbance to overtake us. Instead, the ancients tell us there is a way to free ourselves from the turbulence of strong feelings or thoughts. We still experience our emotions and mental processes, but we remain resting in a quiet, still center without so much energetic dispersion or stagnation. Some mental traits are more ingrained than others. You may have inherited certain ways of looking at the world from your current culture, your parents and guardians, or even generations before that, but you can clarify your mind through specific practices and habits that we explore throughout this book.

Healing the Spirit and Transforming the Heart

The realm of spirit or soul is the most refined feature of your being and another avenue to support yourself. Like the other aspects of self we've explored, this stratum also requires our attention and care if we wish to be fully integrated and healthy. In yoga, this realm is associated with the *vijnanamaya* (wisdom body) and *anandamayakosha* (bliss body). Some traditions associate this territory with something outside of ourselves. However, the spiritual nature I'm referring to lives inside each of us and does not rely on external forces. In this context, our spiritual nature doesn't have form; instead, it is closest to what we call consciousness or awareness. This layer of your being is what determines how you connect with yourself and others and how you relate to your life. It is the sparkle in your eye, what inspires and enlivens you, and what holds the blueprint for your true path in life—your Dao. While we can use the term *soul* to describe this particular aspect of our reality, it's important to mention that in Eastern traditions, it implies something a little different than our Western understanding of the term.

The ancient Daoists called this part of us Shen, which has two uses. Shen can refer to a kind of awareness linked to each organ, or to the "big" Shen that resides in the Heart, which is the source of each aspect of spirit connected to the organs. Nowadays, *Shen* is usually translated as "mind," but as an overarching concept, it is the force that makes us conscious and refers to various facets of the human psyche, emotions, feelings, thoughts, and insights that *live* in our bodies.

When speaking of your spiritual nature, it's helpful to remember that there is virtually no separation between the different layers of your being—whether physical, energetic, emotional, mental, or spiritual. Sometimes, this concept is difficult to understand. We're so used to thinking of the body in a reductionist and mechanical way. However, the body is not simply a collection of physical matter. It is deeply intertwined with our thoughts, emotions, spirituality, and ancestral history. Within this view, the vitalizing forces of willpower, imagination, compassionate action, insight, awareness, intention, and appreciation roam freely within our tissues and organs. In recent years, Western medicine has begun to research and recognize the relationships between mind, body, family history, and environment, but it has only started to scratch the surface. There is so much more depth (already articulated in holistic systems) that modern, conventional medicine has yet to uncover.

In TCM, there are five expressions of spirit or types of consciousness (*Wu Shen*) linked to our organs and the Five Elements: *Zhi*, *Hun*, *Shen*, *Yi*, and *Po*. Each has its own nature or personality that contributes uniquely to your overall psychosomatic and psychospiritual makeup. The *Hun*, or "ethereal soul," is associated with the Wood element and Liver; the *Shen*, usually translated as "spirit" or "mind," with the Fire element and Heart; the *Yi*, translated as "intention" or "thought," with the Earth element and Spleen; the *Po*, or "corporeal soul," with the Metal element and Lungs; and the *Zhi*, translated as "will" or "volition," with the Water element and Kidneys. Your Shen, or spirit, both informs and is informed by the other spheres of your being. An imbalance in this aspect of yourself is often an underlying cause of physical, energetic, mental, or psychological disorders.

Similar to all other aspects of your being, there are many ways to sustain and promote harmony with this subtlest interior sphere. Consciousness dictates how we behave and feel, so working with these energies can help us dance with life and turn it into a creative and conscious act. You can deliberately cultivate and support the quality of your Shen using internal practices like meditation or contemplation, but as you'll see when we look at it more deeply in Part Two, your Shen comes alive as you heal and develop all the other parts of yourself as well. From the perspectives of Chinese medicine, Daoism, and yoga, the more whole and integrated we become, the more we can transform from an identification with a small sense of self into a more expanded view. As this happens, we develop our spiritual qualities, and our emotions and mental states morph into virtues that serve the greater whole. As we work to heal or develop this aspect of being, we're able to live more intentionally and find intrinsic meaning—two essential states that lead to more vibrant health for ourselves and the entire planet.

The primary thing to remember is that all of these realms of being—physical, energetic, mental, emotional, and spiritual—coexist; these worlds within are intimately connected. The ancient wisdom traditions teach us that each shade or texture of experience we encounter is another opportunity to know ourselves in a deeper way. Employing techniques that address each interwoven realm of experience will offer the strongest possibility for health, self-understanding, and ultimately spiritual growth.

—

PART TWO

THE
SEASONS
&
ELEMENTS

SPRING
SEASON
&
WOOD
ELEMENT

FOUR

SPRING STIRRING &
THE WOOD ELEMENT

and I allowed myself
to be astonished
by the great
everywhere
calling to me
like an old
and unspoken
invitation,
made new
by the sun
and the spring,
and the cloud
and the light.[13]
—DAVID WHYTE

We begin our exploration with the Wood element, a time of rapid growth, creativity, and renewal. Like tender shoots of early growth in spring, the Wood element is a time of Yin to rising Yang. Wood symbolizes the miracle of making something out of energy and matter, such as plants transforming sun and soil into living structures. This vigorous impulse toward movement and birth is present in all life. It is the fresh energy that animates creeping vines, the spiral unfurling of fern fronds, the flow of sap, and the start of green buds. You may remember that earth-based traditions show us we can understand ourselves by looking at nature. In our bodies, the energizing quality of the Wood element is expressed as the need for motion and exercise and in how our strong and pliable tendons and ligaments hold our body together and make it move. In the metaphor of life's journey, the Wood element is the young adventurer setting out on their path, determined and full of energy. They may encounter tribulations and obstructions, but their task is to keep their vision clear and learn to flow with the tensions of life rather than be hindered by them—much like the strong fibers in plants keep them flexible and able to adapt when encountering powerful winds.

Trees and all plant life clearly represent many characteristics of the Wood element. The dynamic upward motion of the wise redwoods and giant sequoias and the shimmering new leaves of the gleaming birch, trembling aspen, and majestic oak display a connection between earth and sky, Yin and Yang. As a transitional element between Water (the most Yin) and Fire (the most Yang), the Wood element holds an essential position of growth and creative transformation within the archetypal life cycle of the elements. Trees are revered in many traditions as symbols of life, learning, and growth. Stories and myths centering around a "tree of life," a "world or cosmic tree," or a "tree of knowledge" are common in folktales, religions, and cultures worldwide. Whether depicted in Christianity, Hinduism, Islam, or ancient Native American, Asian, Egyptian, Celtic, Norse, or Greek mythology, trees are seen as sacred. In some myths, these trees provide knowledge, and in others, they bestow eternal life in the form of fruit. In Daoist mythology, for example, trees that grow peaches every few thousand years are said to impart immortality to whoever eats them. In other stories, trees are protected by supernatural spirits and are said to join heaven, earth, and the underworld through their spreading branches and roots.

Within Chinese and Daoist philosophy, the vital energy of the Wood element signifies a fresh start, manifesting in the seasonal cycle as the promise and awakening of spring. Spring often begins with fits and starts and can be a little erratic at times, but like a dawn chorus of songbirds comes alive, it brings active energy and revival. After the challenge of cold weather and dark winter storms, an inner zest returns, and the natural world awakens from its slumber. In old Celtic and pagan traditions, the goddess Brigid, most closely associated with the early spring celebration of Imbolc, is said to invigorate new life at this time by spreading her green cloak across the barren winter land. Mountain snow begins its annual melt, revealing an underbelly of fresh growth; rivers run and swell; and sticky, resinous poplar buds fill the air with the distinct sweet, warm scent of earthy amber and honey. Just beyond my home, the evening air fills with the loud croaking of mating frogs, and the early morning fields are spotted with bright crocuses, daffodils, foraging robins and rabbits, and young deer.

Something vigorous is coming to the surface in the natural world. Throughout the winter, potential energy has been latent, buried deep in the earth, and now, as spring bursts forth, there's a natural impulse to create. I love pushing seeds into the slowly warming soil this time of year, envisioning and planning for the natural and nourishing beauty to come. The herbalist Judith Berger calls this seasonal transition "quickening." She says,

> And what is the name of this force that makes its way into the body rhythm of the animals and wakens them from months of dreaming, that pierces the ruminating dark with the light touch of the sensuous dawn, that makes us toss restless, when we had been so cozy in our warm beds, for winter's end? The name of this power is desire. The desire of life itself for new life, the unavoidable yearning of the dark for its bride of light. And this desire has a heat, and this heat causes a stirring, and the stirring causes a quickening, which causes a flickering flame to wake the bodies of creatures . . .[14]

The season of expanding light is a time of movement, fertility, and revelation; it's a season that supports us in sloughing off the old and outworn and in creating and embracing new growth. The Wood element represents possibilities, the living vitality within that is endlessly creative.

The increasing light of the spring season is celebrated as a special period of earth awakening in many cultures. The *Nei Jing* states, "[T]he three months of spring, they denote effusion and spreading. Heaven and earth together generate life; the myriad beings flourish."[15] As the land bathes in new shades of green, the ancient Celtic tradition of lighting evening bonfires on Beltane represents the sun's power to clear away the darkness of winter and renew the world. Many modern springtime customs commonly practiced in the West most likely originate from ancient earth-based traditions and festivities. During the vernal or spring equinox, a time marking the emergence of longer days and shorter nights, Ostara is thought to have been celebrated in pre-Christian Europe. Named after the Germanic goddess Eostre (and most probably the Greek goddess Eos), Ostara was considered the goddess of spring or dawn and represents the promise of fertility and new beginnings. It is interesting to note that Christians observe Easter at this time, which shares etymological similarities with Ostara. Old traditions like egg painting and hunting, as well as imagery involving mythical hares or cute bunnies, all center around rejoicing in new beginnings and procreation.

Perhaps the most powerful symbols of new beginnings during spring and the ability to be reborn after death or darkness are beliefs and mythological stories involving resurrection. In many ancient agrarian societies, tales of rising after death symbolize spiritual awakening and the promise of new beginnings to come. Christians honor Easter as the time when Jesus, after being brutally humiliated and martyred by oppressive and authoritarian forces, miraculously rose again. In ancient Mesopotamia, the mother goddess Ishtar was given the water of life and allowed to rise after winter in the underworld. In Greek mythology, Persephone returns to the living world in the spring, bringing with her life and the promise of abundant growth. These stories and beliefs all point to the archetypal pattern of the Wood element as it relates to renewal. After periods of struggle, misfortune, and even death, energy will eventually begin to stir and rise again; Wood represents this birth and movement toward something new and alive on the horizon.

The Wood element phase invites us to find clarity around our direction, strategize for what is to come, and creatively move forward with our highest vision. It is a time to renew what is stale and plant or give birth to something fresh and new. When we plan, respond, engage, and grow with imagination and vigorous determination, we are most certainly inspired and empowered by the Wood element's energy. This is the part of us that desires change, the aspect that can rise above or beyond even the most nefarious or difficult of obstacles. Just as plants push upward and start to open during specific times, so do we. Like the stretching of young spring plants, growth and movement are essential for all living things, including humans. Without continual momentum, we become stunted and depressed, never fulfilling our true potential. However, when we lack skillful, focused, and intentional growth, the chaotic winds of change simply bend and shape our direction without any input from us.

It's vital that our direction and vision, linked to the Wood element, hold a certain quality of heart-centered openness within them as we grow. We must stay connected to our wonder rather than becoming too forceful with our desires or direction. In Daoist philosophy, the Wood element has similar characteristics to those of bamboo: its smooth shoots are hollow and empty, flexible yet incredibly strong. Just as the stalks of bamboo need strength *and* bendability, we do too. When working with all of this inspired action, the key is to balance the desire to move forward with a sense of grounding and higher purpose rather than a no-holds-barred determination or aggression. This way, our understanding of destiny and direction is not wildly out of control; it stays internally connected and malleable while reaching toward the light.

WOOD IMAGERY AND LANGUAGE

Sprouting plants and buds
Green moss
Bamboo forest
A circle of cedar trees
Weeds
An eccentric artist
A lively dance floor
Sunrise
An architect

A green traffic light

An archer

A soaring eagle

The adventurer

An argument

Creative play

Dreamtime

A growing child

ENERGETICS OF WOOD CHART

Season	Spring
Yin organ	Liver
Yang organ	Gallbladder
Tissue	Sinew/Tendon
Sense organ	Eyes
Emotion	Anger
Direction	Upward
Sound	Shouting
Climatic influence	Wind
Taste	Sour
Color	Green

SEASONAL SELF-CARE FOR SPRING

As spring arrives, you may feel an inner vitality returning after the cold, dark months. To support the body-mind this time of year, aim to shed the stagnation that may have built up over winter and invite more movement and lightening qualities. Here are a few general suggestions for balancing your lifestyle during the season of stirring and renewal.

> During spring, energy gradually moves up and out, and our focus can shift from being internal to more expansive. Ask yourself, "How am I feeling stuck? What needs to shift so that I can grow?"

> Spring energy builds slowly and can fluctuate. In Chinese medicine, it is a time of Wind—an unpredictable, quick, and erratic energy. To stay balanced, it requires both forward momentum and rooting down, so increase activity bit by bit.

> Daily exercise that emphasizes aerobic activity is best now. Try going for a brisk walk or bike ride, and add movements that increase circulation into your yoga and movement practice.

> Get creative! Dance, paint, sculpt, or draw. Use your imagination to access the vibrant energy of spring.

> Spend time in nature and places that are green (the color of the Wood element). Go for a walk or hike in the forest and open your senses to your environment. Soak in the feeling of growth and expansion. Your Wood element is renewed by being and bathing in beautiful outdoor spaces.

> Focus on regulating your sleep. Wake up earlier, enjoy the extra morning light, and avoid sleeping during the day. Classical TCM texts advise us to make sure we're sleeping between approximately 11 P.M. and 3 A.M. This is because the organs of the Wood element— the Liver and Gallbladder—are more energetically active during that time. You might discover this if you experience a "second wind" late at night when your creative juices start flowing. You can also pay attention to your dreams, which hold special Wood element importance.

> In spring, you may find that you have the desire to start a project or plan a new goal—and the physical and creative energy to get started. What visions and dreams are surfacing for you? What are you nurturing, and what do you feel ready to create?

SPRING STIRRING KITCHEN MEDICINE

During spring, frozen moisture begins to thaw, and Yang Qi rises. Just as the natural world cleanses and comes alive in spring, our bodies and minds do too! In Ayurveda, we say *kapha dosha* increases, which can feel heavy, damp, and cold. In TCM, we support the Liver by moving stagnation and promoting the harmonious flow of Qi. If we're not careful, early spring can be a time when we feel tense, stuck, and lethargic or experience excess mucus and spring allergies.

As spring emerges, food choices should focus on fewer rich winter foods and more mildly warming, simple, light foods. This focus will help you clear stagnation built up from winter and support detoxification. Spring can still be cool and variable, so as with all seasonal suggestions, it's important to make changes gradually throughout the season rather than all at once. It's also a great time to choose foods and herbs that support your liver and help your body cleanse. You'll find a more in-depth discussion of this in Chapter 5. Use these suggestions to maintain good health in your kitchen during spring:

> Eat lighter and less. If you live in a temperate climate, continue eating plenty of cooked foods, but slowly add more fresh and raw foods near the end of spring.

> Increase warming, aromatic, pungent, and energizing spices with a little kick to support your metabolic health and balance the heavier, cooler, and wetter qualities of this time of year. Try mustard seeds, chilies, black pepper, and ginger. If you experience Heat in your body-mind, opt for mint or fennel instead.

> Enjoy green foods and foods that move Qi upward and a little outward—like sprouts, chives, shoots, and leafy greens—to mimic the movement of Qi in the spring.

> Use bitter-flavored foods like arugula, asparagus, artichokes, dandelion greens, kale, broccoli, bitter melon, or romaine lettuce. A small amount of slightly sour food like citrus or dried fruit can also be helpful.

> Don't eat late at night and don't eat if you're not hungry. If you consistently have a low appetite, try a fresh gingerroot tea about thirty minutes before meals.

> Limit heavier foods like fried foods, oily foods, dairy, excessive protein, nut butter, and excessively sweet foods as they cause too much congestion during this season.

> Herbal medicines at this time of year should move your Qi and support your liver, gallbladder, and digestive functions by cleansing and strengthening them. Use herbs like dandelion root (*pu gong ying*) and stinging nettle to nourish and move Liver Qi and Blood. I commonly recommend the formula Free and Easy Wanderer (*Xiao Yao San*) to patients who are stressed and tense in the springtime.

As you can see, the Wood element is all about renewal, growth, and flow. We can work with these Wood element energies in nature and receive their gifts in many ways. Seasonal food and self-care choices are a good place to start, but there's so much more to discover about Wood. Remember, each element has a resonance. Once we understand the subtle energy an element represents, we can apply this understanding to all aspects of our lives, including the physical and subtle body, which we'll explore next, and our emotions and spiritual life, which we'll delve into in the next two chapters.

ORGANS OF THE WOOD ELEMENT

In Chinese medicine, the organs in the body that connect to renewal and direct the energy of the Wood element are the Liver and Gallbladder. The physical liver is located mainly on the right side of the abdomen, partially protected by the rib cage. It is the body's largest internal organ, and with hundreds of functions, it supports almost every other organ. We can't live without it! The liver's main physical job is detoxification. It breaks down and processes practically everything the body doesn't use. Specifically, it filters and metabolizes substances in the blood. As blood moves through the liver's tissues, the liver extracts and breaks down toxins, aiding in their removal and excretion. It is also responsible for the metabolism of fats, carbohydrates, and proteins, synthesizing amino acids and cholesterol. Finally, the liver stores minerals, blood, and some vitamins. It also produces bile, which it sends to the gallbladder, a small organ beneath the liver. The gallbladder stores and secretes bile that the liver produces, which helps during digestion, particularly of fats.

The Wood element and the Liver and Gallbladder also have energetic functions. Remember, when we speak of the organs in Chinese medicine, we refer to a whole system, not just the physical organ. Energetically, the Yang organ of the pair—the Gallbladder—collects, stores, and excretes bile, similar to how it is understood in Western medicine. If this function is impaired, you may experience digestive issues or a feeling of distention in your upper abdomen. In TCM, the energetic Gallbladder also controls our sinews (tendons and ligaments) for movement. When one of my patients is stiff, has a history of straining or tearing their tendons and ligaments, or tends to be too mobile due to a lack of stability, I always make a note to assess their Wood element. Healthy Gallbladder Qi ensures that our tissues can literally jump into quick and decisive action.

Your energetic Liver stores Blood, which circulates throughout your body, enlivening your tissues and providing deep nourishment, oxygen, and moisture. While the Gallbladder controls your tendons and ligaments, your Liver nourishes and moistens them with rich and lubricating Blood, allowing movement. In Chinese medicine, we aim for the body to have enough Blood—*and* Blood that's full of energy; it should be plentiful and nutrient-dense. In Chinese medicine, Blood is more than the fluid that pumps through veins and arteries. It is a very dense form of Qi and also a vehicle for Qi. Good-quality Blood forms through a complex energetic process between the digestive system and the Lungs, Heart, and Liver. We make it from digested and assimilated food with the help of Jing (which we'll explore in Chapter 16), which is partially housed in the bone marrow. Energetic Blood is a Yin-like substance. It has a grounding influence on your body-mind, and it contributes to breast milk and menstrual blood. When your Blood doesn't provide enough nourishment or isn't flowing adequately, your mind and spirit don't have an anchor to allow them to settle and rest, and you'll have trouble sleeping or feel anxious.

Healthy Blood supported by good Qi circulation feeds your skin, nails, eyes, hair, and tongue. When your Liver Qi and Blood are healthy and flowing smoothly, you'll look vibrant and feel energetic and flexible. If your Blood lacks deep nutrition or doesn't flow smoothly, you'll feel tired, spacey, and ungrounded and may be in pain. You may also have brittle nails, numbness in your extremities, dull eyes, and pale or purplish hues on your skin or tongue akin in some ways to the symptoms of anemia. When I have a patient with these symptoms, a blood test may not identify low iron, but a Chinese medicine diagnosis can still help me detect that the quality or amount of Blood is low.

The Liver also moves vital energy called Ying (nutritive) Qi to all of your tissues and organs via blood vessels and meridians, moistens your eyes, and contributes to tears. If I have a patient who complains of dry, red, or itchy eyes or general vision issues, I assess the health of the Wood element overall. Vision applies to our physical sight but also to our ability to dream and envision our future. We'll cover that in Chapter 6.

The most essential function of this system, though, is the smooth flow of Qi. Just as the general in an army ensures everything is moving harmoniously, the Liver always maintains even movement, which is critical because Qi's motion drives all processes in the body-mind. Its natural flow aids everything from our ability to digest food to the easy movement of Blood through our arteries and veins to our ability to release emotions. Qi flow even helps us get creative and have a sense of direction. When the smooth flow of Qi is impaired, pressure builds up, and you may experience migraines, digestive problems, pain, depression, anger, and even severe heart abnormalities. Qi flow (and therefore the movement of Blood) is also essential to the uterus and breasts, so concerns about fertility, menstrual issues of all kinds, and breast pain are usually linked to the Wood element too. Ultimately, we feel tense, stuck, and stagnant without healthy Wood element organs. If there is a lack of relaxed and balanced flow—physically or emotionally—we look to the Wood element system to reestablish movement and harmony.

WOOD ELEMENT MERIDIANS

Just as each element has a corresponding season and associated organs, it also has specific energetic pathways that circulate Qi and Blood. The Liver Sinew channels begin at the top of your big toes and ascend to the front of your inner ankles and up your inner legs to your groin. The

Liver's primary channels also encircle the genitals and run up the front of the abdomen to the ribs. The Gallbladder Sinew channels begin at the top of your fourth toes. They traverse the sides of the body from the outside ankles, knees, and hips with branches to the sacrum, ribs, and breasts. Then they ascend the neck and the sides of the skull, passing behind the ears, with branches to the sides of the cheeks, nose, and eyes. From there, they terminate at the top of the head.

To support these channels and subtler meridians associated with the energetic Liver and Gallbladder, and the Wood element in general, we can choose specific movements and yoga postures that target the tissue that wraps and weaves around the structures of the side body and inner leg. Anatomically speaking, many people are tight along the side of the body where the Gallbladder channels run, yet they remain weak in the inner legs where the Liver meridians lie. When the Wood element is stressed, this pattern can become more obvious, leading to tight outer hip, buttock, neck, and upper back muscles, as well as headaches, especially on the side of the head.

Sensing the Wood Element Channels and Organs in Supta Padangusthasana II (Reclining Big Toe Pose II)

Lie flat on your back on a firm but soft surface, like a blanket spread over a yoga mat. Exhale deeply a few times and allow your bones and muscles to drop. As you relax, feel the heaviness of your hips, legs, and feet; let go of any holding and release your body toward the floor. Visualize the energetic pathway of the Liver channel along your inner legs and groin, and the Gallbladder channel along your outer legs, hips, side torso, and the sides of your neck and skull. Feel one side of your body and then the other. Is one side more tense or lax? Scan the sides of your body and notice if or how your legs fall out to the sides. It's common to have excessive drag toward external rotation due to fascial restrictions in the side body and weakness in the inner legs. If you're having trouble feeling this, interlace your fingers and place your palms behind your head. Use your hands to pull your head off the floor so you can peek down at your feet. To what degree are your feet pointing outward? Quietly observe in a nonjudgmental way how this pattern shows up in your body.

Next, bring your awareness to your physical liver and gallbladder organs. Green is the color we associate with these organs of vitality and Wood Qi. If it helps, you can place your hands on your abdomen, just below your diaphragm and right of center, where these organs live. As you breathe, simply intend to be present and feel. The organs in this area can become stagnant and conflicting, or they can pulse together harmoniously. Imagine a vibrant, forest green color permeating your energetic Liver and Gallbladder with energy. Visualize this color for 5 to 10 breaths. When that is complete, relax your focus and roll to one side.

Now you can sense these meridians and energetic organs in a yoga posture like Supta Padangusthasana II. To begin, place a bolster or cushion beside your right hip. Draw your right knee into your chest and loop a strap around the sole of your foot. Extend your leg straight up and pull gently on the strap to add some resistance. Straighten your left arm out to the side and ground your left hip to the floor. Then, open your right leg to the side to rest on the bolster. Feel how this movement creates sensation in the inner leg and groin and outer hip, where the Liver and Gallbladder channels run.

If you're comfortable there, you can once again use the color visualization with your internal organs. Stay for 1 to 2 minutes, attuning to these pathways and organs. Switch legs and try the pose on the other side.

FIVE

GROWTH & SMOOTH FLOW

Now in the spring I kneel, I put my face into the packets of violets, the dampness, the freshness, the sense of ever-ness. Something is wrong, I know it, if I don't keep my attention on eternity. May I be the tiniest nail in the house of the universe, tiny but useful. May I stay forever in the stream. May I look down upon the windflower and the bull thistle and the coreopsis with the greatest respect.[16]

—MARY OLIVER

So far, we've explored how the Wood element manifests in nature and the seasons and how it is represented in the body through the organs, tissues, and meridians. Now we'll look at how the ebb and flow of this spirited energy causes us to go out of balance and some practices to help us revitalize this system.

WOOD ELEMENT QI STAGNATION

Mental stress causing tension and stagnation is among the most frequent Wood element concerns I encounter in my clinical practice. Nearly all instances of what we normally call "stress" are at least partly linked to the Wood element, whose role is to facilitate the smooth flow of Qi—and emotions are a form of Qi. You'll generally experience a fairly even temperament when this function works, but when it does not, emotions won't flow and can build up and become toxic. Additionally, when we experience stress, it's common to seek comfort through substances like alcohol, prescription medications, or marijuana, which further deplete and stagnate the Wood element in the body and mind. In Chapter 6 we explore how the smooth flow of Qi contributes to emotional control, direction, and regulation, especially for anger. Essentially, if we don't learn to feel our emotions and express them in healthy ways, they get stuck, congest our system, and lead to Qi and Blood stagnation. If stagnation sticks around for too long, the energetic Liver will generate excess Heat as it attempts to find balance, leading to concerns like inflammation, frustration, headaches, or constipation. If emotions lack smooth flow or are repressed, the body-mind can also eventually "give up," and stagnation will turn to depression.

In Chinese medicine and Daoism, emotions arise from the internal organs; you may remember from earlier chapters that if we deny or repress them, they become one of the primary causes of disease. This is because when emotions don't transform, they cause agitation in the Heart-Mind; when the Heart-Mind is not settled, we're not able to act in alignment with our Dao or true path in life. Whether you're feeling overwhelmed and having difficulty scraping by or are tense about a relationship or an upcoming deadline, if you're feeling stressed, chances are your Qi isn't flowing. Qi stagnation and stress are highly prevalent in many of our lives, but stress is not a disease in and of itself. It is a natural reaction to life circumstances. Some stress helps us stay motivated and is even healthy, but unfortunately, many people live way beyond a manageable level. The explanation of the Water element in Chapter 17 looks at how chronic stress is extremely depleting. Be sure to read that section if you feel stuck in a stress response or are experiencing fatigue from long-term, low-level stress.

Qi circulates throughout the entire body and interacts with all the elements and organs, so when stress and Wood element issues cause Qi to stagnate, many systems in the body can suffer. If your Wood element is directly implicated, you'll likely experience general Wood element symptoms related to your energetic Liver and Qi and Blood stagnation, such as premenstrual syndrome (PMS), headaches, depression, or a feeling of distension in your body. You may have a difficult time releasing mental and emotional frustration and instead remain narrowly focused, intolerant, bound up, and tense.

Habits to Move Stagnation

If you want to ease stress, strengthen your Wood element, and move stagnant Qi that has built up, here are a few habits to implement right away:

> Consider the load you're placing on your liver. Stay away from foods and substances that are congesting, like highly processed and deep-fried foods, and limit recreational drugs. While alcohol and marijuana may temporarily ease Liver Qi, allowing you to feel better in the short term, long-term use stagnates Qi and clouds your vision (the spiritual aspect of the Wood element, which we'll explore in the next chapter). Many commercial beauty products that do not contain natural ingredients, as well as prescription and over-the-counter medications, also burden the liver, so reduce or limit them when you can.

> Eat a diet of high-quality, healthy oils, such as omega-3 fatty acids from avocados, flax and chia seeds, and fatty fish. Eat colorful vegetables, especially cruciferous, bitter, and green ones, such as broccoli, brussels sprouts, dandelion greens, and kale.

> With guidance from an herbalist or practitioner, add herbal medicines like milk thistle and bupleurum (*chai hu*) to heal and support your liver and its functions.

> Opt for a simple seasonal cleanse at least twice a year. A detox or cleansing program doesn't have to be extreme or intense. Instead, use it as a time to simplify your routine and diet. Try eating lighter and less, and eat simple food combinations with plenty of steamed greens for a few days. Or try a broth fast if you are especially congested. If your digestion is strong, add a fresh green vegetable juice daily or do a green juice fast.

> Drink one teaspoon of unrefined apple cider vinegar added to a glass of water daily for a week or two. If you experience Heat in your body, try the juice of one lime in water instead.
> Get moving. Make sure to get moderate to vigorous exercise daily. Refer to the practice section in this chapter for more ideas on specific postures and movements to try.
> Track your rhythms. An even Qi flow relates to all the cycles of your life. Notice how your body adjusts to the seasons, times of day, and aging. Track your sleep and menstrual cycle to determine whether your Qi is flowing or stagnant. Make sure to get adequate sleep every night. If your menstrual cycle is irregular or delayed, you most likely have an imbalance and would benefit from working with a practitioner to restore harmony.
> Spend time planning goals that feel good and envisioning your future. Make a digital vision board or create one using old magazines. Build a detailed list that breaks down your plans and dreams into bite-sized tasks. Make a point of crossing things off the list and celebrating as you achieve your goals.
> Pay attention to your level of busyness. A simple schedule and fewer to-dos support the smooth flow of Qi. People who tend to be stressed a lot usually have too many plans on the go. Say no to more tasks when you can, and aim to balance downtime and work.

INNER AND OUTER VISION

The eyes are the sense organs for Wood. Our Wood element connects our physical vision and our emotional and spiritual visionary capacity.

I don't think many people would argue that we use our eyes too much and too often in our modern world. Beyond the damaging, often violent content we consume, we live in a culture that is simply transfixed by the wonders of visual stimulation. Many of us spend hours every day looking at our computer screens and phones, which can create agitation and restlessness in the mind, resulting in eyestrain, stress headaches, anxiety, and insomnia, all of which I regularly see in my medical practice. While the causes of these conditions are almost always multifactorial, we know that the blue light many of our devices emit has genuine effects on the brain and its production of melatonin, an essential hormone needed for good sleep, rest, relaxation, and circadian rhythms.

Visual input stimulates thinking. Consider how rapid eye movements suggest a mind that is restless or distracted. Even in sleep, the movement of our eyes indicates greater brain activity and vivid dreams. In Ayurveda, the eyes are the realm of *agni* (fire); *alochaka pitta* is responsible for generating visual impulses. Pacifying the eyes softens the mind's tendency to constantly project and identify with form. For this reason, yoga practitioners will often relax their eyes to calm and clarify the mind. As they deemphasize physical sight, they encourage *inner* sight associated with the mystical third eye. This energetic center is inside the skull, along the midline of the lower forehead. It is considered an entryway into higher states of perception and a significant area of study and inquiry. This vortex of energy correlates with the physical location of the pituitary, hypothalamus, and pineal glands, which are important for many hormonal functions, including the release of melatonin mentioned earlier. There is also an acupuncture point in this area called *Yin Tang*, or "Hall of Impressions," located on the forehead between the eyebrows. If you've been receiving acupuncture for any time, you may have already experienced this! It is one of the most common points, as it is very effective at calming the mind and spirit, helping to ease agitation, restlessness, and insomnia.

Sight, externally and internally, is one of life's most incredible offerings. When we see clearly, vivid visions and beautiful colors inspire us, and the movement of the Wood element is unhindered, drawing us forward. When seeing remains clear, we perceive the truth; our view is broad and all-inclusive. We see our path and can walk it with determination. Too much visual stimulation affects our physical sight and our ability to access internal visualization and dreaming. We're drawn outward into the world because of desire fueled by empty visual cues, not inner seeing. In yoga, we pacify the eyes and aim to slow the movements of the mind to counteract this.

I often teach *pratyahara*, or sense withdrawal, in my classes to support the eyes. I love handing out the classic Iyengar head wraps (similar-looking to an elastic bandage you would use for a sprained ankle) and asking students to wrap their heads and cover their eyes for meditation. This method blocks visual input and has a gentle compressive effect on the skull, which students find very therapeutic. You can accomplish a similar effect at home by wearing an eye mask during Savasana (Corpse Pose) or other restorative pose.

In the next practice, we'll explore another way to support the eyes and the piercing quality of the outer and inner sight available to us with gentle gazing.

Trataka Practice

The traditional practice of *Trataka* entails gazing steadily. The ancient yoga text *Hatha Yoga Pradipika* describes it as "looking intently" and refers to it as eradicating all eye diseases and fatigue.[17] Considered a *shat karma* or *kriya* (a cleansing technique) in yoga and Ayurveda, it also has a balancing action. In another ancient text, the *Gheranda Samhita*, Trataka is even considered a way to cultivate clairvoyance. In any case, this therapeutic practice helps relieve eye tension and can be an effective antidote to headaches due to eyestrain.

Trataka is the practice of settling and concentrating the mind on a single point to withdraw from the outer world and attain complete absorption. During the practice, the gaze and concentration are placed on a single object, often a candle flame. You can try a similar practice by gazing at the moon or, as I do sometimes, watching the reflection of light on a body of water. I enjoy doing this practice in the early morning or the evening. Do Trataka alone or before other forms of practice. If you've had any form of eye surgery or suffer from migraines or glaucoma, consult with your health care provider and an experienced teacher before trying this practice. No need to take off your glasses if you have myopia.

Choose a dark room free from artificial lighting and air drafts so the candle has minimal flicker. Start by practicing for 15 minutes.

Place a candle at eye level about two to three feet in front of you. Sit in a comfortable meditation posture, relax your body, and encourage an upright spine. Close your eyes and begin with a short meditation to calm and settle yourself. Take a few slow, soft breaths and aim to arrive in the present moment. We'll begin with a few simple eye movements.

Keeping your eyes closed and your head still, look up and down three times with just your eyes, returning to the center at the end. Next, look right and left for three rounds, returning to center when finished. Finally, circle your eyes in one direction and then the other three times. Rest in the center once you're done. Relax any tension in and around your eyes and collect your attention on your breath. Softly breathe in and out.

Now open your eyes and light the candle in front of you. Return to your meditation posture and gently gaze at the candle flame. Focus your awareness on the brightest part of the flame. Do not blink, but do not force your effort; keep your gaze unwavering in a delicate way. Steady your attention and soft gaze on the object of concentration—in this case, the candle flame. If your eyes become tired, you can lower your eyelids slightly.

Eventually, you will notice your eyes tearing or feel the need to close your eyes. When you do, keep your attention on the visual impression of the flame at the back of your eyelids. Draw awareness toward the general area of the Yin Tang point on your lower forehead between your eyebrows. Continue witnessing until the image fades, then continue your internal gazing and rest in the space of awareness for the remainder of your session. After the practice, you can rub your palms together and gently cup your eyes to encourage further relaxation. Avoid rubbing your eyes if they are tearing; tears in this situation are thought to result from a detoxification process; simply dab tears away with a tissue.

Releasing Stagnation with Wind Pool

Did you know the muscles at the base of the skull (suboccipitals) connect directly to the eyes? Maybe you've felt this connection if you've spent too much time staring at a computer screen. It's common to have both eye and neck strain coupled. Let's explore this with a short practice.

Begin by lying flat on your back on a firm but soft surface, like a blanket spread over a yoga mat. First, we'll locate the acupressure points called Wind Pool (*Feng Chi*). Find them at the base of your skull below the occipital bone in the small hollows on either side of the spine (between the sternomastoid and trapezius muscles). Begin by placing your thumbs at these locations. Close your eyes and try to move your eyes up and down and side to side without moving your head. Do you feel how the suboccipital muscles respond to eye movements? If you're under stress, Wood element energy can blow upward and lodge in the neck and trapezius at or around these points.

Next, place the base of your skull on a soft ball or the edge of a yoga block. Soften your eyes and roll your head from side to side, putting pressure on the tender spots along the occiput (base of the skull) for 3 to 5 minutes, or however long feels good. Use this to clear tension and address headaches, neck pain, sinus congestion, and eyestrain. In my acupuncture practice, I also use these points to activate the whole Gallbladder meridian and release Wind. You may remember the pathogen Wind from Chapter 2; it's especially prevalent in spring (Wood element season) and can manifest as an unsettled nervous system, dizziness, spring allergies, headaches, spasms, itchiness, pains that move around, and a lack of clarity.

Similar to the practice of yoga, a significant component of working with acupoints is inner listening. If you're grounded and present, you may notice subtle changes or a natural time when the area feels complete. Experiment with lengths of time and pressure until you find what works for you. Once you've finished putting pressure on the points, rest on your back for a minute or two, observing any feeling of circulation or warmth.

PRACTICES FOR BALANCE

We can work with the Wood element system in many ways through yoga and meditation. First, movement in general is extremely useful because it helps Qi circulate, and the Wood element is responsible for the smooth flow of Qi in the whole body. All movement improves physical and mental flow, which helps the Wood element do its job. That's one of the reasons why exercise is so beneficial when we're feeling stressed and tense. In particular, creative and spontaneous movement like dance encourages the free-flowing nature of the Wood element's energy. To support Wood, approach your yoga practice with a spirit of play—creative sequencing and music can help accomplish this. If you teach, try telling a joke during class to lighten the mood.

Twisting postures bring a fresh sense of aliveness to the body and mind because of their ability to "unwind" tension and free up stagnation that are so common with Wood element imbalances. We'll also explore side bending and poses that stretch the inside and outside of the leg and outer hip where the Wood element meridians run. My favorite group of postures for this purpose are what we generally call "hip openers" in the yoga world. Before diving into a few poses in this category, let me say that for good hip health, we need all kinds of movement—not just "opening" (which usually refers to external rotation and flexion). If you're a practitioner who regularly stretches or "opens" the hips with poses like these or others such as Eka Pada Rajakapotasana (Pigeon Pose), be sure to include practices that strengthen the outer hips, hamstrings, and inner thighs as well.

Unwinding Yin Somatic Twist

Lie flat on your back on a firm but soft surface, like a blanket spread over a yoga mat. Bend your legs and ground your feet about hip distance apart. Place your arms out to the sides in a T position, with your palms facing upward. On an inhalation, drop your knees to the right without lifting your feet off the floor (roll onto the inner edge of your left foot and the outer edge of your right). As you twist, pin your left shoulder to the floor—don't let it lift. Sometimes this movement with the legs is called "windshield wipers," but it's a little different than what you may be familiar with. Move rhythmically with your breath. (You'll notice we're moving *into* the twist on the in-breath, not the out-breath, as is commonly practiced in yoga). As you come back to center on the exhalation, feel your whole body settle and drop before taking the movement to the left. Slowly go side to side five to seven times, feeling your body and any subtle releases as you return to center.

On the next round, as you drop your knees, stay in the twist longer for this final version—anywhere from 1 to 4 minutes, as long as it remains comfortable. Pause and relax, feeling the twist of your spine and obliques and any "massaging" or squeezing in your abdomen and internal organs. As you stay in the posture, let out a sigh if it feels good. Sighing can help reset your nervous system if you've been under stress and is one way the body naturally releases stagnant Liver Qi. As you return to center after the longer hold, once again notice your whole body settling into neutral before moving to the other side.

Restoring Flow with Hip Openers

I've highlighted the Yin Yoga postures of Shoelace, Square, and a variation of Sukhasana (Easy Pose) in this practice. Depending on your body, you may prefer one pose, so experiment and see what works for you.

Begin seated on a small cushion or folded blanket to create a slight anterior tilt in your pelvis. To get the effect in the hips and groin we're trying to achieve, stack your knees with your feet out to the side for Shoelace or stack your shins for Square. When practicing with your knees stacked, it's helpful to pull your top thigh back a little so your hips are almost even. In Sukhasana, which may be the most accessible variation for you, cross your shins out in front of your body with each foot under the opposite knee. Feel free to use the support of a blanket under one or both knees as you set up any of these postures.

From this position, fold forward without collapsing into your diaphragm (if you have a history of kyphosis—rounding of the upper back— keep your spine upright). Bring your hands to the floor and press gently to rock your weight back into your hips until you feel pressure or tugging in your inner groin and outer hips where the Liver and Gallbladder energetic channels run on either side of your body. Be careful not to put too

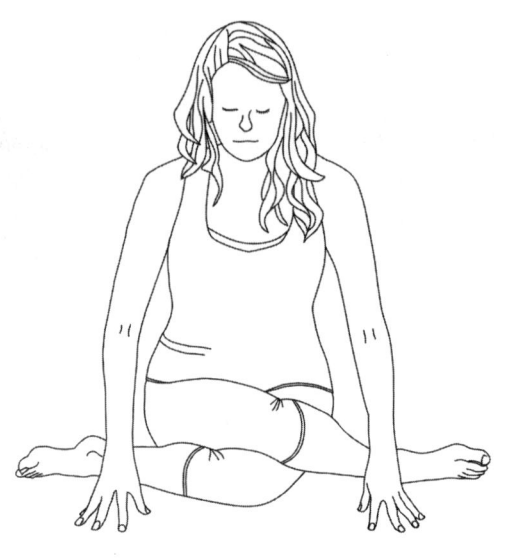

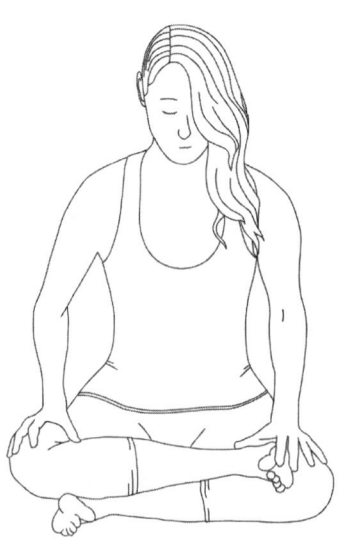

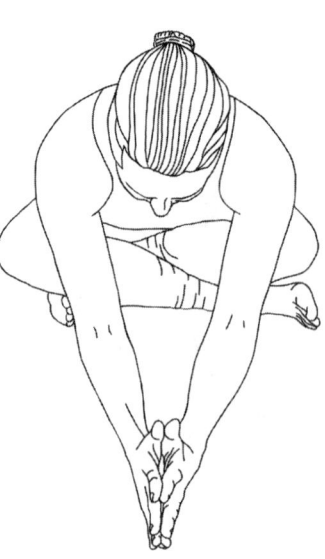

much pressure on your knees. If you experience pain in the upright posture or are avoiding forward bending, try practicing these poses on your back by grabbing your ankles or the soles of your feet.

Stay in the pose for a few minutes. To release, sit up and use your hands to guide your legs out; rest back on your hands. You can also perform a countermovement by gently twisting or doing a windshield-wiper movement with your lower body and legs.

Adho Mukha Svanasana (Downward-Facing Dog Pose) Outer Heel Push

Step back into Adho Mukha Svanasana. Set your feet to the width of your yoga mat, bring your toes slightly in, and push your heels out. Lift onto the balls of your feet and reach your heels and sitting bones skyward. If you have tight hamstrings or a tight lower back, bend your knees and lift your sitting bones, while drawing your lower back into a concave shape. From there, press your heels toward the floor, mainly focusing on your outer heels as you lengthen your side waist. Repeat this movement a few times, lifting your heels and then pressing your outer heels down. Finally, hold the pose for ten to twenty breaths; feel any lengthening and spreading along your lateral legs and torso where the Gallbladder channels run.

Parighasana (Gate Pose) Variation and Utthita Parsvakonasana (Extended Side Angle Pose)

These postures stretch the sides of the torso, reducing congestion and encouraging space and length along the Gallbladder channels, especially in the outer legs, oblique muscles, and side ribs. They also target the Liver channels if you feel a pull in your inner leg and groin.

The name of our first pose, Parighasana, comes from the gatelike shape formed by the body. Start in an upright kneeling posture, with your hips over your knees, facing the long side of your yoga mat. Step your right leg out to the side so your foot is pointing away from you and toward the top of your mat. Make sure your heel is in line with your left knee. Place a block on the inside of your right foot. Inhale and raise your arms out to the sides at shoulder height. Exhale and bend sideways toward your right foot. Place your right hand on the block. Keep your left hip aligned over the knee on the mat. Reach your left arm overhead, creating a side stretch through your torso. Turn your abdomen away from the floor and feel a lengthening in your spine. Hold the pose for several breaths, feeling the expansion along the side of your body. Inhale as you return to the starting position, and repeat on the other side.

Next, we'll practice Utthita Parsvakonasana. Come to standing, step your feet wide apart, and place your left foot parallel to and pressing against the baseboard of a wall. Bend your right knee, gently rolling your outer knee open. Ground your whole right foot, and press the outer heel of your left foot toward the floor and wall. Lean over and place your right hand on a block, a chair, or the floor next to the inner arch of your right foot. Reach your left hand overhead so your side body is long. Feel how this creates a ripple of sensation and activation up the sheathing of your outer leg and the side of your torso, where the Gallbladder channel runs.

Sense into your right leg. As you bend your right leg into the side angle position, sense engagement or a tug in your inner leg where the Liver channel runs. Stay for 30 seconds to 2 minutes, breathing and sensing. Switch legs and try the pose on the other side.

In this chapter, we explored how the Wood element commonly stagnates and some habits and practices to harmonize Wood. In the next chapter, we'll examine its subtle aspects, including emotional and spiritual imbalance and associated practices.

SIX

THE CREATIVE IMPULSE

Trees are poems that the earth writes upon the sky.
—KAHLIL GIBRAN

Just as the grand fir, hemlock, and spruce spread upward toward the sunlight, the emotional energy of the Wood element wants to rise up and move toward what it desires. It will thrust itself forward against obstacles to get what it needs. It's responsible for our assertion—the energy that fuels growth is the same energy that drives our vision, creativity, plans, and goals, as well as our feelings of anger. The Wood element relates to many shades of anger, including frustration, annoyance, intolerance, impatience, hostility, and rage. These manifestations all have the same fundamental energy; they want to push ahead unimpeded, just like the branches of a great tree press upward, seeking the sun. When the natural surge of energy inherent in the Wood element is healthy, we can start something new. We know what our dream is, and we can create a plan, set goals, and take decisive action that will get us there.

You will remember that the Wood element is responsible for the smooth flow of Qi. Anger is associated with the Wood element because when Wood element energy doesn't flow or get what it wants, the buildup creates tension and friction. Think about it: when you have a strong opinion or desire about what direction you want to go, it's easy to get frustrated when you encounter resistance or blockages. It's like banging your head against the wall; you want to move forward, but you can't. That's the essence of anger. The fiery nature of anger can be uncomfortable—and for good reason. Without careful attention, rage can burn out of control and turn to hostility and hatred, destroying everything in its path. Or it can be repressed and smolder within, leading to self-rejection, shame, or depression. Whether it's external or internal, anger without appropriate tending turns into violence, aggression, or hatred and, of course, can be very harmful.

Many of us are socialized to think anger is always a negative emotion and that being a good person means you should never have strong feelings and reactions like rage or frustration. Sometimes I see this attitude in the yoga and meditation world. Commercial depictions of such practices often idealize detachment from worldly concerns or exclusively emphasize "feeling good" as the ultimate goal of practice. Because of this, it's easy to think we must deny or ignore the more challenging aspects of our experience if we want to be "spiritual." When this happens, yoga and meditation become self-soothing mechanisms rather than vehicles for self-awareness or transformation. There's nothing wrong with caring for ourselves and wanting to feel good, but there are also gifts in exploring and working with the so-called negative emotions like anger.

When we're healthy, we don't ignore or eliminate anger. The energy of anger has its place. When we encounter a barrier that elicits a strong reaction, we receive a noteworthy message from within. Anger can be an essential defense and an expression of our boundaries. It sends a signal that something is wrong and points us toward what is central in many wisdom traditions—our conscience. In its rarefied state, anger is pure energy that helps clarify our values. When refined and used correctly, it provides great power and sharp insight into what direction or action we should take, and it allows us to see what we need to do. When anger positively empowers us, it can be a potent and creative force for change, transforming our fury into loving action. We'll explore how to do that later in this chapter.

The thing is, even when our Wood element is healthy and things are flowing smoothly, challenges still happen; it's a natural part of life. You can see this in plants when they begin their circuitous route upward in the springtime. Just as new seedlings need to break through hard ground and twist and turn around any number of obstacles, we, too, face challenges to our movement and growth. As you walk your unique path and try to bring your heart's vision into reality, you will naturally encounter difficulty and resistance. When I assess the emotional health of the Wood element, I look at how an individual handles these setbacks. Rather than getting angry or being too timid to act, are they able to retain a strong vision and direction but adapt when they need to? When we have a healthy Wood element, we're able to see the bigger picture and meet adversity and constraints with flow and flexibility. We realize that obstacles provide opportunities for greater understanding and creativity.

Just like the Qi stagnation we explored in the last chapter, when our Wood element is out of balance, sometimes the smallest of setbacks can cause tension and stress to accumulate and intensify. We get frustrated and unable (or unwilling) to find a path forward. For instance, some people will angrily and endlessly fight against a limitation without first considering whether there are alternative ways around it. Others will immediately claim defeat and give up. Both reactions keep us stuck and unable to move. In my clinical practice, I often see folks who have long-standing Qi stagnation from built-up anger that manifests in myriad stress conditions, such as depression, headaches, teeth grinding, and pain disorders. As with all emotions in Chinese medicine, if anger goes on too long, is extreme, or isn't expressed, it will cause imbalance. Ultimately, instead of giving in to frustration, reactive anger, or total apathy and collapse, we must connect with our hearts and get the energy moving again. When we do that, we have access to the true virtue of the Wood element—a state of visionary action rooted in love, which we'll explore in the next two sections.

THE SPIRIT OF WOOD

In Traditional Chinese Medicine, each of the Five Elements has a quality of spirit or type of awareness that contributes to its overall characteristics. For the Wood element, the type of consciousness is the Hun, sometimes called the "ethereal soul." The Hun is the part of us that can see things from many perspectives and apply them in ways that will satisfy the Heart. In classical texts, the Hun is ghostlike, airy, and mystical. It comes and goes like the wind. Whereas the Wood element itself connects to our physical sight, the Hun connects to our inner vision. It helps us see our path more clearly; it's involved with our imagination and regulates our dreams while we sleep. Like the trees are a link between the earth and sky, the Hun joins our vision to our earthly existence and vice versa.

In the Five Element model, Wood lies between Water below and Fire above. As a junction between the Water and Fire elements, the Hun ties together our most profound potential (Water) and the Heart's highest purpose (Fire). Wood energy wants to move forward; the Hun is what helps us do that. It's both a dreamer and an action-taker. Lao Tzu suggests what can happen without the guidance and perspective of the Hun:

> The unyielding army cannot prevail.
> Unbending trees are felled.
> The great unyielding belong below,
> The pliant and tender above.[18]

Through a delicate and creative dance with the ever-changing circumstances of our lives and outer world, a healthy Wood element and Hun help us easefully grow, adapt, and change direction, while serving our visions and plans.

The spiritual gift of this type of consciousness emerges not only when we're able to make decisions, dream, and plan, but when we can also transform those visions into something more focused on, and aligned with, the good of all. Rather than trying to control things for personal gain, this aspect of our spirit and psyche can guide us toward our most benevolent aspiration. In yoga and Buddhism, we call this compassion, or *karuna*. When the Hun is in its most elevated state, anger transforms into hope and becomes the outer momentum in which self-centered motivations fall away. The Hun's perspective and vision, coupled with its compassion, allow us to lead others, stand up for what is right, and constructively transform even the most difficult circumstances. Without this higher quality of the Wood element, it's easy to slip into unproductive outrage or depression when we encounter difficulty, as we saw earlier, or just push forward solely focused on our own desires at the expense of others.

We can look to many inspiring change agents who epitomize these higher qualities of the Hun, such as visionary leaders who imagined, stimulated, and guided movements throughout history using nonviolent direct action and a radical philosophy based on love. Some of these well-known leaders include those involved in the women's suffrage movement, such as Elizabeth Cady Stanton; the anti-apartheid activist Nelson Mandela; the civil rights leader Martin Luther King Jr.; and Malala Yousafzai, an activist for female education. Mahatma Gandhi, the man who led the successful campaign for India's independence and inspired civil rights movements worldwide, said he followed two primary vows (*yamas*) on the eight-limbed path of yoga—*ahimsa*, literally translated as "restraint," "nonviolence," or "nonharming," and *satya* (truth). These guidelines helped Gandhi overcome and evolve an oppressive ingrained system without succumbing to hate or violence. The moral discipline of ahimsa reminds us that the welfare of all beings is equally important. We are bound together by the fabric of life; harm done to one is harm done to all. All of these visionary warriors saw inequity and used the intensity of their outrage to incite positive change. They transformed their frustration, resentment, or deflation into care, and when encountering seemingly insurmountable challenges, they used their energy to stir loving momentum in their communities.

The poet Dinos Christianopoulos says, "What didn't you do to bury me, but you forgot that I was a seed."[19] Just as the buried seed uses Wood element energy to push through hard-packed ground, we can use this energy to effect change. Those who see injustice or pain and operate from intention dictated by the Heart to find solutions have become a seed for change; they have transformed anger into compassionate action. Many of the Buddha's profound yet simple teachings highlight this sentiment: Hatred, greed and delusion are never overcome by aggression. Instead, we surmount them with love. Channeling dreams of a better future and taking action based on loving-kindness are desperately needed today. To have the energy and capacity for this, we need to do the inner work required for our outer work to take hold, as we explore next.

INSIGHT AND COMPASSIONATE ACTION

Much of our modern-day culture is based on pathological systems of oppression and domination over people and the earth. There's no doubt, then, that strong thoughts and feelings in response to these painful, hard truths can arise when we turn toward the complex and demanding circumstances surrounding us. Whether we look at social, political, or environmental troubles, when we honestly confront the many pressing issues of our time, we are bound to react with resistance or moral outrage. While tangible work in our communities is essential, we must also learn to relate skillfully to our own reactivity. We must distill powerful emotions into positive forward momentum rather than getting stuck in them or letting them drive us. Remember, Wood element energy wants to move. When our Wood element is out of balance, we experience *nonproductive* anger toward ourselves or others, or we feel defeated and give up. However, when our Wood element is healthy, we have the capacity to transform the energy of anger by connecting to our Heart, and in this case, it turns into a flexible vision, ideally for the benefit of all beings.

In Buddhist philosophy and practice, we can look to the bodhisattva, who epitomizes this quality. *Bodhi* is the Sanskrit word for "awake," and *sattva*, in this context, means "being." Joined, they refer to a person who bravely lives in this world with an inclusive and wise heart. The peaceful warrior of the Wood element understands that the welfare of all beings is equally important. When we embody this sentiment in our lives, we both exemplify the spiritual virtues of a healthy Wood element and strengthen our Wood element at the same time. We can practice this aspiration daily by connecting to a more expanded worldview, remembering that all beings suffer and seek happiness. We can also dedicate the merit of our activities to the benefit of others, whether in our family unit, workplace, or larger community.

The beautiful, many-handed Buddhist bodhisattva of compassion, Avalokiteshvara (also called Guanyin), symbolizes this resolve. The mythical tale of this bodhisattva goes like this: One day, after diligently and vigorously trying to relieve the suffering of many other beings, Avalokiteshvara looked around and realized there were still multitudes of people suffering she had yet to reach. In a moment of discouragement and despair, her head shattered into many pieces. To help, the Buddha responded and gave her eleven heads so she could better hear the world's cries. However, when she attempted to extend herself toward those cries, there were simply too many, and her arms broke into pieces as well. Once again, the Buddha came to her aid and bestowed upon her a thousand arms with an eye of wisdom in each palm so that she could see the world's suffering and spread her loving compassion to all. Each of us attempting to walk the path of practice will sometimes lose connection to our most profound wisdom and compassion. We all face burnout, disappointment, loss, and struggle, but the question as it relates to the virtue of the Wood element is whether we will give in to these obstacles or allow them to strengthen our resolve, like Avalokiteshvara.

So how are we to embody this wisdom in our own lives? First, we need to step back and understand how and why we get blocked. The Wood element helps us do that through a refined type of inner seeing—or insight. The Buddha skillfully outlined the practice of *vipassana bhavana* (insight meditation) to accomplish this clarity of perception. *Vi* means "into" or "through," and *passana* translates to "see" or "perceive"; vipassana is the act of seeing into something in a special way. *Bhavana* comes from the root word *bhu*, which means "to become" and describes mental cultivation. Therefore, vipassana bhavana is the cultivation of the mind to see things clearly. During vipassana meditation, we use mindful attention to observe the ever-flowing movements of the mind, body, and experience to understand the true nature of our reality.

Some days when you sit down to meditate, you may discover that you're actually quite riled up and distracted. You're not alone. In fact, it's common when we practice mindful awareness to find that states like judgment, comparison, attachment, aversion, desire, and fear are what keep us from seeing clearly. These obstacles, as we all know, are unavoidable. The ancient yoga text Patanjali's Yoga Sutras lists nine common obstacles that can get in our way: illness, apathy, doubt, neglect, laziness, indulgence, lack of clarity, instability, and lack of a sense of progress. In the Buddhist canon, we can look to five classic hindrances: sensory desire, aversion, sleepiness, restlessness, and doubt. These barriers interfere with a natural opening of the heart and clarity of mind, which we need if we want to embody the virtues of the Wood element and be agents for positive change in our world.

Sometimes, these states are really apparent, showing up as endless distractions designed to tempt us. At other times, they sneak into our quiet presence like thieves in the night, slipping into our minds and luring us away from presence by exploiting our moods and personal tendencies. During yoga or meditation practice, you might initially experience this as restlessness or desire: "Maybe I should finish my shopping list, clean out that closet, or grab a cookie from the kitchen rather than continue." If you manage to maintain your focus and resolve, you may eventually experience doubt ("Is this even working?"), aversion ("I hate that annoying clock. I wish it would stop ticking."), or a sense of pride ("I'm such a good meditator/yogi!"). The key is to see these visitors clearly and allow them in without reaction. Although they are a fundamental part of the untrained mind, not even the most experienced meditators are immune.

To work with such distractions during our practice, we can turn the hindrance into the object of meditation rather than just an external diversion. We certainly don't want to avoid or suppress them (that would be a form of aversion), and we don't want to react or respond to them immediately either, as that would just strengthen the hindrance itself. As we direct our consideration toward the distraction, we can observe how it operates. Does it change? What are the sensations, emotions, or feelings attached to it? In this way, what once obscured our focus is now helping us to strengthen and deepen our awareness.

It's still possible to have a stable and free mind—even while encountering these disruptions—as long as you remember that every hindrance provides an opportunity for insight and self-understanding. Just as we can distill outrage and use it skillfully to fuel compassionate action, any obstacle can supply fodder for our practice. Distractions are nothing more than a passing state of mind; you'll notice that even the most challenging things will change. Eventually, that craving for a cookie subsides, your doubt relaxes into a moment of calm abiding, or that sense of aversion or pride shifts into a little more wakefulness.

This technique is fundamental because it supports us in dealing with and being present for difficult mind states in practice and life. For example, when we feel anger rising, we can mindfully watch how it affects our thoughts and feelings before trying to determine a good way forward. Wisdom, compassion, and insight naturally arise when we see what is happening *and* how we relate to it before acting out. Suppose we don't take this first step of mindful attention. In that case, we risk acting out of violence, irritability, or another unacknowledged feeling or emotion rather than from a place of genuine understanding and awareness. By seeing clearly and becoming familiar with our inner struggles, we come to know the roots of our suffering and how to remain equanimous when encountering changes or challenges, no matter their type. All of this aids us in being more effective when we can and do act personally or for the collective good.

When we recognize, accept, and open ourselves to where we get stuck, we often discover that loosening around our struggle happens naturally. To deepen your understanding, use the following suggestions during reflection or when you feel triggered by an intense reaction.

HEALING THE WOOD ELEMENT

> Acknowledge your feelings with kindness. When encountering strong emotions, the first step is to recognize their presence, soften, and let things be without judgment. Like Qi, emotions want to move, but it's vital first to pause and ask yourself, "What is the particular flavor of the feeling or emotion I'm experiencing? Where am I caught? How do I experience this in my body? Is this feeling directed at someone else or myself?" Kindness and compassion naturally arise when we contact our suffering. To support this natural arising of care, it may help to offer yourself a few quiet phrases like "Yes," "I allow," or "This too," while placing a hand on your heart or abdomen. Remember, working with your feelings is not a cognitive exercise. Listen quietly, observe bodily sensations, and practice offering care toward whatever arises.

> Cultivate curious, nonjudgmental attention. As you observe your emotions, sensations, and feelings, notice how you relate to and

react to whatever is present. Investigate how you may be holding on to something or pushing it away. We humans have a general tendency to reject what we judge unfavorable, to cling to what we regard as positive, and to "zone out" during more neutral experiences. All these responses lead to suffering because we lose the opportunity to experience the richness of the entire present moment. The great news is that noticing these tendencies weakens them. Rather than reacting to what you encounter, ask yourself, "What is this emotion or feeling showing me? What is asking for my attention? What does the part of me that is struggling most need right now?"

> Aim for flexibility and focus on what you can control. As we discussed earlier, when faced with change or challenge, our resistance, rigidity, and lack of adaptability often cause the most stress, inappropriate anger, and Qi stagnation. At times, our strong emotions give us messages that a boundary has been crossed, and a specific change is needed. It's essential to listen to that. However, at other times, you may need to consider how you can change your outlook. We can't always control our outer circumstances, but we can control our responses. Ask yourself if you can see the situation in a new, creative way or direct your assertive energy toward a different goal or direction, such as your own self-care.

> Let go when you can and find your bigger vision. The Wood element is healthiest when we loosen our grip on life and allow it to flow without so much identification with a personal "self." If you often find yourself irritated or cynical, a reminder not to take yourself and life so seriously may be necessary. That can be a tall order if you're used to being angry, disappointed, or shameful, but over time, it gets easier. Spend time daydreaming and exploring your grandest and most imaginative visions. If you are holding a grudge against yourself or another that you're ready to work with, try the forgiveness practice that follows here. The Wood element has an incredible capacity to renew by conjuring up new plans and possibilities and initiating Heart-centered actions.

Working with Aversion in Yin Yoga

During Yin Yoga, we hold passive yoga postures for extended periods. In this practice, we'll use our yoga posture as a place to watch our natural tendency to avoid or move away from unpleasant things—what we call the "hindrance of aversion or ill will" in yoga and meditation.

Begin by choosing one of the Hip Opener variations in the practice section of Chapter 5. You're going to stay in this pose for a little longer than usual as a way to begin investigating how you deal with aversion.

Set up your posture with any props you need and settle in. Provided your body feels like it is in a safe position, open your attention to include whatever thoughts and sensations arise. Are you feeling restless or bored? Are there moments when aversion creeps in? Get curious and notice. Maybe this position is feeling really good, and you want to extend the time in the pose because it stirs up pleasant thoughts or feelings. If you're unsure whether any mental state is surfacing, just stay with the sensation and allow it to expand and change with time. The longer you hold the pose, the more intense the sensation will probably get. Take your time and observe how things feel and what thoughts, emotions, or reactions arise. No need to try to interpret; just stay with the pure experience itself.

As time goes on, you can start noticing any reactivity you may be feeling. A longer-held Yin Yoga pose is a perfect place to watch the mind wanting to escape the moment! Aversion appears as any number of annoyances, discomforts, or preferences: "I don't like this exercise," "It's too stuffy," "It's too cold!" Often, aversion shows up as an angry, fearful, judgmental, or bored mind state. As we explored earlier, the aversive or angry part of you can be an influential teacher. First, you must get to know it. Whichever tone of aversion you experience, sit with it. Feel its texture, and open to it softly and mindfully. Don't try to avoid it or push it away, even if you dislike it or wish it were different somehow. What would it be like to welcome this feeling, sensation, or thought and give it a generous place at the table?

As we develop mindfulness, contentment grows. Agitation, boredom, or fear lessen and become more manageable when our presence is strong. By watching our tendency to want things to be other than they are, we begin to notice our attachments. Like all other hindrances, aversion is conditioned by circumstances and prone to the laws of nature, including the truth of impermanence. Whatever is bothering you will change. Breathe and stay with it.

If the particular type of aversion you're experiencing is challenging to be with entirely, it's helpful to cultivate the qualities of care and compassion. You may want to offer yourself some soft words of kindness as you stay with your discomfort.

Stay in the posture for 2 to 5 minutes, then switch the placement of your legs and repeat on the other side. When you're done, slowly release and rest for a minute or two.

Forgiveness Practice

In this practice, we'll explore a guided meditation, first focusing on asking for forgiveness and then offering ourselves forgiveness. Forgiveness can be difficult, especially if you feel angry or betrayed about something. Still, it is an essential step in healing the Wood element and stepping into its higher expression of benevolence and compassionate action.

Find a quiet place in nature where you won't be disturbed. You could bring a natural offering with you, like a flower, to give to the earth. Find a comfortable sitting position by arranging a little room around you that's free from leaves, sticks, or stones. Most importantly, find a place where it's possible to relax and maintain the focus of your attention. We'll begin as always, settling into breath and body awareness. As you drop into your meditation, relax and notice your breathing for a few cycles.

Once you have established a stable place of arrival, think of a time you caused harm to another person through your words or actions. Picture the situation and imagine the pain and hurt the other person may have felt. Allow yourself to feel your own pain and shame. Keep the situation in mind, and when you're ready, silently ask for forgiveness. You could say something like, "I know I hurt you. Please forgive me." Allow whatever feelings or thoughts are present without judgment. Open to the possibility of forgiveness.

Next, turn your attention to the natural world around you. Stay connected to the times you may have caused harm. Ask yourself if there are ways you have wronged another or maybe even Earth herself. You can place a hand on the soil beneath you or on a nearby tree as you contemplate. As you consider this question, imagine any deeds you wish to be forgiven and lovingly absorbed by the earth. If you've brought an offering, you can place it on the earth as a simple gesture of connection and care. Earth doesn't hold grudges and will always embrace you when approached with reverence. Once again, you might say a few words, such as, "I'm sorry. Please forgive me." After phrases like that, pause and return to quiet meditation, allowing yourself to feel.

Now turn your attention to yourself. Consider any ways you have harmed yourself, either in this same situation or another one. Visualize the circumstances surrounding the event and feel any pain or regret you're holding. When you're ready, ask yourself for forgiveness. You could silently say, "May I forgive myself," or "I see the pain I caused, and I forgive myself." End your meditation with some moments of quiet awareness. Return to your body and breath, and simply be, allowing any thoughts or feelings to arise.

The Wood element distinctly expresses the creative energy of life. All growth relies on this powerful force. As we move from the darkness of the Water element to Wood, we emerge into the light. It is a time of *beginning*. We've explored how its rising Yang energy is manifest in nature and in our bodies and minds. When balanced, the qualities of Wood are rooted yet malleable. In the Five Element cycle, Wood's roots are nourished by Water, and its fibrous material feeds Fire. In our next section we'll dive into the season of sun and the radiant power of the Fire element.

SUMMER
SEASON
&
FIRE
ELEMENT

SEVEN

SUMMER THRIVE & THE FIRE ELEMENT

For the sun is the honey of all beings and all beings are the honey of the sun. The consciousness of the sun shines in the eye of all beings. It is the never-ending, the creator, the all.[20]
—BRIHADARANYAKA UPANISHAD

Following the new growth of the Wood element, energy now reaches its zenith with the most Yang element of the five: Fire. Fire is also an essential part of life. Think of how the glowing energy of the sun is at the heart of our world; without sunlight, life on earth would cease to exist. We have entered the season of maximum expression and function. Fire's enthusiastic drive and intrinsic luminosity are contagious, inviting us all to thrive and express ourselves. We can feel its resonance in summer sunflowers, shooting stars, the twinkling of fireflies, and heartfelt laughter. When in harmony, its expansive and warming nature energizes all things. The Fire element is an active force in our bodies, contributing to all sorts of necessary metabolic processes like digesting proteins and fats, pumping blood, and maintaining hormones that regulate mood and temperature. On a psychospiritual level, the Fire element stirs our hearts and encourages intimacy. It also symbolizes our awareness; in many early yogic and Daoist teachings, the sun represents consciousness. The blooming energy of Fire helps us live in alignment with our true nature. It blesses us in enjoying life through relationships, community, a sense of playfulness, presence, and a willingness to share our vibrant selves.

The natural world reflects Fire's invigorating and dynamic vibration with showy, colorful, and riotous displays. You can see it in the flickering sunlight on a hummingbird's flashy green back or the spirited blush of opening flowers, their radiant color and aroma attracting attention and admiration. Flowers are a perfect metaphor for the Fire element because they represent a plant reaching its full potential. In its flowering, a plant offers its seed, pollen, and fruit to the life cycle, graciously beginning a new generation. Similarly, the very tangible flames of fire are needed to revitalize life in the natural world. Periodic fires help forests stay healthy; some burns are necessary for good regeneration, and humans have been conducting controlled burns for ecological health for thousands of years. As a fire sweeps through a forest, it increases soil fertility, releasing stored nutrients held in dead and decaying plants, and it opens the otherwise latent and pitch-sealed cones of trees such as the great lodgepole and jack pine. As the cones open, their seeds spread and create new growth. Fire is intensely transformative—for good and bad. Wildfires, of course, can also lead to massive destruction. As I write this chapter, many places around the globe are battling devastating and unprecedented summer wildfires, a sign that the Fire element is out of balance in our world today. The fierce and all-consuming nature of Fire tells us it requires careful maintenance and respect if we are to harness its power and honor its place in the cycle of things.

According to Chinese and Daoist philosophy, the heightened energy available from the Fire element relates to the bright and enlivening summer season. Like the rising flames of fire that naturally spread up and out, the long days and warm air of high summer feed body and spirit and fuel outward activity and celebration. The risk of spring frost is long gone, and now, for a brief moment, the natural world opens its heart wide and shares its grace, vibrant color, and juicy fruit with the world. The swifts and swallows swooping through the skies and the lengthening evenings signal that it's finally time to fling the windows and doors open, shed our protective coverings, and stand in the warmth of the sun. Like enjoying a perfect cherry tomato plucked on a warm day, summer is a time to fill our hearts and minds with abundant beauty and delight. With its scent of strawberries, lemon balm, and sweet peas, summer is a time to languish in the long days, take pleasure in loved ones, and appreciate the Yang power of light and heat.

The other seasons of the year are a little darker and quieter, so folks tend to get overly eager for summer's sultry solar energy and long-lasting twilight when they come; the pull to connect with others, enjoy gatherings, and play outside is strong. This is the energy of Fire! Fire helps us refuse anything that might shut us down or limit our pleasure. It also helps us remember a deeper connection to humanity as a whole. Richard Wagamese touches on this feeling when he writes,

> It is love itself that brings us together. This human family we are a part of, this singular voice that is the accumulation of all voices raised together in praise of all creation, this one heartbeat, this one drum, this one immaculate love that put us here together so that we could learn its primary teaching—that love is the energy of Creation, that it takes love to create love.[21]

With a well-adapted Fire element, you can have healthy boundaries and still be vulnerable, openhearted, and generous, as well as experience human connection as a form of communion with the Divine.

Like an eagle drifting on a mild breeze or a monarch butterfly floating through the meadows, I always try to savor my time outdoors during this season. There's nothing quite like a summer barbecue, beach fire, picnic in the park, or late-night dip in the lake with family and friends. During this season, I especially relish waking early and making medicine with wild roses, which are plentiful in our area during the early summer. Wildflowers, and especially the delicate pink blooms of wild rose, always remind me of the Fire element season growing up with my little sister in the prairies of Canada—how we spent long summer days building forts, lying on our backs watching the clouds, and picking brown-eyed Susans in the ditches and fields beyond our home.

Since ancient times, humans all over the planet have celebrated this season and elemental energy with festivities marking the fieriest day of all—the summer solstice—when earth's axial tilt is closest to the sun and the day is the longest. For those of us with a Celtic background, chances are our pre-Christian ancestors lit bonfires and hosted parties to revel in the power of the Fire season. During midsummer, the Germanic celebration of Litha honors the light of the sun and the rhythms of nature inherent in the wheel of time. The *Nei Jing* describes it this way: "The three months of summer, they denote opulence and blossoming. The qi of heaven and earth interact and the myriad beings bloom and bear fruit."[22] With its joyous energy, Fire kindles warmth in our hearts, sustaining us even during grim times and the inevitable darker days.

The Fire element represents a lightness of spirit, but it's so much more than that. When tamed, Fire reveals our inner knowing and radiance—the untouchable emptiness of our Heart-Mind, which we'll explore in Chapter 9. In Ayurveda, when we refine the Fire of the mind, the positive aspects of Tejas—pure intelligence, brightness, and piercing clarity—are revealed. In Daoist and Chinese theory, when we settle the Fire of the Heart, we illuminate its pure nature and discover it can hold all things in its openness—our elation, our despair, our wonder, and our sorrow. Just like the steady beating of the Heart, the present moment is constantly happening, becoming, and being, and we are not separate from it. The illuminating nature of Fire provides warmth and clarity and helps us be self-aware and present in this very moment. The spiritual gift of Fire helps us access the Heart's highest knowing, even amid chaos. When we do that, we can more easily surrender to our inner truth and follow our Dao. We step into our right place among it all and find the birds, the bees, the supermarket, the traffic jam, and the trees all have a space for us.

FIRE IMAGERY AND LANGUAGE

Volcanoes
Buzzing bees
Candles
Hot peppers
A summer festival
Red roses

Electricity
Our inner child
High noon
A charismatic entertainer
Sunbathing
A bright smile
An optimist
An explosion
A bed of hot coals
Passionate sex
A phoenix

ENERGETICS OF FIRE CHART

Season	Summer
Yin organ	Heart and Pericardium
Yang organ	Small Intestine and San Jiao
Tissue	Vessels
Sense Organ	Tongue
Emotion	Joy/shock
Direction	Outward
Sound	Laughing
Climatic influence	Heat
Taste	Bitter
Color	Red

SEASONAL SELF-CARE FOR SUMMER

During summer, the key is finding the right amount of Fire. It's a great time to be open and experience joy and expansion, but as the weather gets hot, temper Heat by slowing down and choosing practices that are cooling. This way, you can rejoice in the vibrancy of this Yang time of year, but by the time autumn comes, you won't be overheated and burned out. Here are a few general suggestions for thriving in summer without feeling agitated or exhausted.

> This is a time to be more extroverted and open to safe and wholesome connections with others. Ask yourself, "How can I improve my relationships?" Build healthy emotional intimacy by speaking from your Heart and practicing loving communication (with yourself and others). Share laughter and cuddles with family and friends. Invite people over for a meal or gathering. Practice selfless service and spend time contributing to your community.
> The key in summer is equalizing outward movement and inner containment. Think of balancing Heat and Cold, action and restoration, relationship and solace, so you can sustain your energy through the season.
> Moderate exercise is best during the heat of the summer. Get your heart pumping, but avoid vigorous exercise and excessive sweating, especially around midday.
> Wake with the sun and rest when needed.
> Enjoy yourself and do what brings you joy!
> Take hikes; get outside and spend time in nature. Enjoy sunshine in the morning and cool walks in the shade.
> Avoid overbooking yourself. Schedule downtime daily.
> Take cool showers, jump in a lake, or try moonbathing.

SUMMER THRIVE KITCHEN MEDICINE

Summer is the most exuberant and Yang time of year. Gather with others to eat a variety of simple, fresh, and seasonal colorful fruits and veggies prepared with care. Now is the time to appreciate your summer garden, visit the local farmers market, prepare dishes that bring you joy, and focus on foods that are calming and balanced. This will alleviate any buildup of Heat and cool the body and spirit.

In the summer, your body craves less food and gravitates toward dishes that are refreshing and light. Bitter and cooling foods are important to counteract the obvious heat of summer, but take care to maintain some internal warmth. Often, summer comes with too many cold foods, like ice cream and iced drinks. Over time, this cold stagnates and can slow digestion. Excess Heat and Yang can cause dehydration and drying in the hotter months, so foods that support Body Fluids and Yin are also required. Follow these general tenets for summertime wellness in the kitchen:

> Eat less and choose lighter and mostly plant-based foods.

> Add in some fresh raw foods like cucumber, celery, sprouts, and salads. (However, if your digestion is weak, it's fine to stick to mostly cooked foods, even in summer).

> Eat cooling foods like aloe, tofu, coconut, zucchini, and mung beans.

> Summer is when we want to support the energetic Heart and spirit. The best way to do this is with a *sattvic* (light, or "pure") diet, which focuses on simple whole foods that are not too stimulating.

> Stay hydrated with water and green tea. Drink coconut water, or add a slice of lime or cucumber to your water for extra electrolytes.

> Cook foods for less time and with more water, such as giving them a quick water sauté, steaming, and blanching.

> Include more bitter flavors, such as leafy greens (dandelion, romaine, escarole, endive), asparagus, zucchini, fennel root, rye, and radicchio.

> Enjoy red foods and sweet, juicy fruits like watermelon, berries, grapes, apples, and stone fruits.

> Use small amounts of warming, pungent foods and herbs. They are initially warming, but ultimately they bring heat to the surface of your body and help you to perspire and cool down. Chilies and cayenne are good choices.

> Avoid alcohol, coffee, and refined sugar; go easy on heavy, oily, or salty foods, including nuts, seeds, meats, eggs, and grains.

> Herbal medicines at this time of year should focus on cooling, calming, and nourishing the blood. Use herbs like chrysanthemum flower (*ju hua*), mint (*bo he*), and Chinese angelica root (*dang gui*). Consult your doctor about the last herb if you're pregnant. If you have trouble sleeping and feel depleted, hot, agitated, and anxious, the formula Sour Jujube Decoction (*Suan Zao Ren Tang*) helps calm the spirit and nourish the Blood.

The enthusiastic nature of the Fire element brings to mind vacations and revelry. We can tap into and harmonize these energies by making seasonal cooking and self-care choices. However, the power of Fire also lives in our bodies and minds. Let's look at the subtle body organs and meridians here and investigate the world of Fire element emotions and spirit in the next two chapters.

ORGANS OF THE FIRE ELEMENT

In TCM, the Fire element relates to four internal organs—the Heart, Small Intestine, Pericardium, and San Jiao. The heart and pericardium are located in the chest, inside the rib cage and a little left of center. They are part of the cardiovascular system, which includes arteries, veins, and capillaries. The heart nourishes (in cooperation with the lungs) the body-mind by continually pumping an enormous amount of oxygen-rich blood (around two thousand gallons a day!) through the vast circulatory system. This function is so important that if the heart stops beating for more than a few minutes, life ends. The pericardium is the outer fibrous layer or sac around the heart. It supports the heart's movement and functions while providing a physical protective barrier between the heart and surrounding tissues.

The small intestine is another Fire element organ; it's located in the gastrointestinal (GI) tract, between the stomach and the large intestine. It receives food from the stomach and continues the process of digestion. The small intestine is where a large portion of the absorption and assimilation of nutrition and fluid occurs. The San Jiao (also called the triple heater/burner) is not recognized in Western anatomy. There is some dispute about what physicality the ancients were referring to when they discussed the San Jiao, but it's widely believed among TCM physicians that it refers primarily to various functions and a *relationship* between organs instead of a specific organ on its own.

The Fire element and its associated organs are not only responsible for these physical duties; they also have energetic characteristics. As with the Western perspective, our energetic Heart governs our blood and blood vessels. Hence, any concern with physical cardiac function and blood circulation, such as hypertension, arteriosclerosis, or palpitations, lies with the Heart. Its ability to circulate blood can also affect our complexion. Maybe you know someone who simply glows? That means their Fire element is strong and healthy. A dull or pale complexion without a rosy luster may indicate a deficiency.

In Chinese medicine, we call the Heart the emperor (I call it our empress; it is a Yin organ, after all). The *Nei Jing* says it is "the official functioning as ruler. Spirit brilliance originates in it."[23] As the monarch of the body, it rules and responds to all emotions and feelings and provides a place for our highest vibrational force—Shen (spirit)—to rest. The energetic Pericardium acts as the Heart's guardian and protector physically, emotionally, and spiritually. The Heart and Pericardium oversee all mental activity, relationships, intimacy, joy, communication, and overall sense of presence, well-being, and pleasure. We'll explore these functions more when we examine the emotional and spiritual aspects of the Fire element in Chapter 9.

The Small Intestine's energetic roles and responsibilities are similar to those of its Western counterpart. In TCM, it's responsible for sorting the pure from the impure during digestion. Any concerns related to the absorption of nutrients indicate Small Intestine involvement. As mentioned earlier, the San Jiao does not have an exact anatomical location, but it does have necessary energetic functions. The term literally means "the official in charge of three burning spaces," which is a nod to its function of regulating and managing the movement of Qi, fluid, and even warm temperatures through the three energy centers called *jiaos* (burners)—the upper chest, midabdomen, and lower abdomen.

Lastly, the Fire element controls sweating, so we want to assess your Fire element if you have either excessive or no sweating. This element also governs the health of the tongue, which includes speech and laughter. When I have a patient who talks a mile a minute, has a speech impediment, or displays some other noticeable trait when they speak, I take special note of their Heart Qi. In TCM, we also look to the tongue for valuable diagnostic information overall. When I see a patient, I ask about their health, take their pulse, and ask to look at their tongue. A person's tongue color, shape, and coating give me clues about their underlying pattern of disharmony. An ideal tongue is pink and moist, with a thin white coating. In particular, the tip of the tongue, which specifically relates to the Heart, and a crack along the middle of the tongue can give indications about the health of the Fire element.

FIRE ELEMENT MERIDIANS

When working with each element, we can identify subtle energetic meridians that link to the energetic organs. The meridians of all four Fire element organs lie primarily along the inner and outer aspects of the arms. The Heart Sinew channels start at the inner (radial) aspects of the little fingers and travel along the palms to the inside (medial side) of the elbows, then to the chest, diaphragm, and abdomen. The Small Intestine Sinew channels begin on the backs of the little fingers and travel up the ulnar (outside) aspects of the arms to the upper back and shoulder blades, then up the neck to the backs of the ears and sides of the face and jaw with branches that enter the ears. The Pericardium Sinew channels begin on the tips of the middle fingers and travel along the palms up the center of the arms to the chest, ribs, and diaphragm. The San Jiao Sinew channels run from the outside (ulnar side) of the ring fingers up the back (posterior aspect) of the arms to the shoulders and neck, with branches to the jaw, tongue, temples, and near the eyes. The primary channels also circle the ears.

To support these channels and subtler meridians associated with the energetic Heart, Small Intestine, Pericardium, San Jiao, and the Fire element in general, we can choose specific movements and yoga postures that target the tissues of the arms, chest, shoulders, and shoulder blades. When Qi flows freely through these structures, we can breathe more freely, and we exhibit more openness and availability—all qualities of a healthy Fire element. However, it's common for folks to display a permanent posture of retreat, with rounded shoulders and a sinking chest. This is often from spending too much time hunched over a computer or other factors like emotional shutdown and constriction. Either way, the Fire element won't thrive if this area remains hindered.

Sensing the Fire Element Channels and Organs in Salamba Setu Bandhasana (Supported Bridge Pose)

Lay a bolster lengthwise in the center of your mat; place a block at one end and a thin, folded blanket at the other. Sit on the bolster and lie back so that your head and shoulders drop toward the floor but the lower tips of your shoulder blades remain on the bolster. Extend your legs and place your feet on the block. Rest your head on the folded banket, but don't compress your neck by using too much height under your head. Soften your throat and bring your arms out to the sides in a T position, palms facing up. Some compression in your back is fine, but if you feel any discomfort, especially in your lower back, use less height (like a folded blanket instead of a bolster) or bend your legs and place your feet on the floor.

Take a few minutes to settle into the pose. This gentle inversion should provide a sense of space in the front of your body while gently increasing blood flow through your neck and throat. Relax your body and notice how it feels.

Next, bring your awareness to the pathways of the Fire element channels. The Heart and Pericardium meridians run along the inner arms and upper chest, while the Small Intestine and San Jiao meridians are at the backs of your arms and shoulder blades. As you rest for 2 to 3 minutes, notice any sensations that are present and invite a gentle, spreading quality through these areas.

Next, bring your attention to your physical heart, pericardium, and small intestine. When healthy, these organs work together cohesively. When out of balance, they can become chaotic and disharmonious. If it feels good, place your hands on your body where each of these organs are located. Most of what we think of as the belly is where the small intestine lies. The heart and pericardium in the chest are almost entirely surrounded by the lungs except for a small area at the front just behind the sternum (breastbone) and in the back near the front of the spine.

Red is the color we associate with these organs of connection and Fire energy. As you breathe, imagine a glowing red color infusing your energetic Heart, Pericardium, and Small Intestine with energy. Feel the fullness in your chest and belly. Stay visualizing this color for 5 to 10 breaths. To exit the pose, soften any focus and roll to one side.

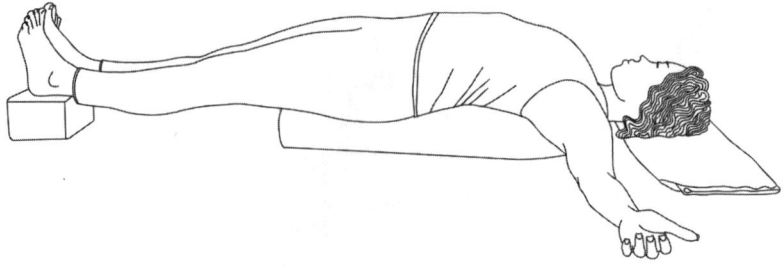

EIGHT

INNER GUIDANCE

[T]here is a place in you where you have never been wounded, where there is still a sureness in you, where there's a seamlessness in you, and where there is a confidence and tranquility in you. And I think the intention of prayer and spirituality and love is, now and again, to visit that inner kind of sanctuary.[24]
—JOHN O'DONOHUE

We've explored the vigorous vibration of the Fire element in nature and the season of summer and how it manifests in our physical organs, tissues, and subtle energetic channels. Fire hums with the mood of togetherness. It's all about fun and connection, but not just connection with others—with ourselves too. Now we'll explore some ways we lose this connection and how we can come back into harmony.

FIRE ELEMENT DISCONNECTION

The Fire element stimulates activity and can be lovely when we're having fun on a summer afternoon. However, just like with all the other elements, we need balance for health. Fire can burn out of control and become destructive if left unchecked. When unrestrained, it can scorch or deplete us; when it's not stoked appropriately, it can fizzle out. Physically, excess Fire can deplete our vital fluids, leading to rashes, breakouts, palpitations, urinary tract infections, and digestive trouble. But in TCM, when it comes to Fire element health, we especially want to watch out for psychological disruptions. This is because our Heart (a Fire element organ) is so closely tied to consciousness. In fact, Eastern systems point to the Heart—not the head or the brain—as the residence of the "mind." Ancient Daoists highlighted this in their calligraphy: the characters for Heart and Mind (Xin) are the same. The Fire of the Heart-Mind contains two intermingling forces—our consciousness or intelligence and our capacity for care.

When the Fire element and Heart-Mind are balanced, we have just the right amount of subtle warmth, which gives us appropriate levels of joy, a sense of belonging, openheartedness, contentment, and clear perception. When this element is healthy, we can even be just a little bit wacky and spontaneous. Folks with a lot of Fire in their constitution know that this human experience is a little wild and can be amusing. It certainly isn't all serious. Generally, this means we also enjoy good sleep and steady energy. We have a sense that everything will work out in a big-picture sort of way; that life is coherent, meaning whatever life we are leading at this moment is aligned with our true nature. It is the light of our Fire element that guides us throughout our lives, so when this system is balanced, we spend less time doing things that don't truly matter to us, and we experience more ease around following our life path or Dao. Because we know who we are and are living in harmony with our true selves, we also attract more fulfilling relationships and are more comfortable with intimacy. Maybe you've experienced a time in your life like this, where you seemed to glow and attract serendipitous connections because you were "right on track." You could say this is the essence of healthy charisma, the kind that only comes from a Fire element and Heart-Mind that are settled and on the correct path in a very deep way.

One of the primary ways we get thrown out of balance with Fire is losing touch with our Heart-Mind—our inner guidance and spiritual self. Like a flickering flame, our Fire can become unsteady, and we end up feeling estranged, dispersed, and disconnected from ourselves and others. When I'm assessing the health of the Fire element in a clinical setting, I look for a few key indicators. Most importantly, I look for whether my patient feels spiritually connected and what their capacity to self-reflect is like. If I have a patient who experiences acute sadness, seems to waver about who they fundamentally are, or lacks insight into their unique direction in life, I take note. I also watch for a steady kind of spiritedness and happiness, appropriate laughter, and even a twinkle in the eye. In Chinese medicine, the glint in a person's eyes signifies the light of consciousness within them. The *Nei Jing* says, "The eyes are the emissaries of the heart. The heart is the residence of the spirit."[25] Dull or absent-looking eyes, or an inability to maintain eye contact, indicates something has gone awry with the Fire element. It could be due to exhaustion, a trauma from which the person hasn't yet recovered, addiction, or mental illness, but it definitely is a cue to assess the Heart-Mind.

If you have a Fire imbalance that involves your Heart-Mind, you'll either exhibit signs of hyper- or hypoarousal. For example, if a person craves overexcitement or experiences anxiety, agitation, stuttering, palpitations, or insomnia, they may have too much Fire or Fire energy that is flaring upward, disturbing the Heart-Mind. When things start feeling too fast and frenzied, it's a sure sign this element is out of balance. If a person feels abnormally cold, overly timid, depressed, disconnected, or resigned, they may have too little Fire. In this case, they need to stoke the embers of their Heart to reignite their passion and love for life. You can see from these two polar extremes that balance is somewhere in the middle. We need some excitement, but too much of it is destructive and, in extreme cases, becomes hyperagitation. On the other hand, when we don't feed our Fire, too little stimulation turns to indifference or apathy.

You may have noticed that many of the pathological symptoms mentioned here are common responses to extreme stress or emotional or physical trauma. This is because even though many systems, elements, and organs are profoundly affected and can become dysregulated during emotional or psychological difficulties, it is our Fire element that is impacted the most when we encounter shock or overstimulation of any kind. When we're resilient enough to return to a baseline of quiet after an exciting or stressful experience, our Fire element is most likely healthy. In Chinese classical texts, the characters linked to emotion include the character for the Heart and indications of clarity and even nourishment. They imply that when emotions are allowed and experienced in a space of calm or stillness within the Heart, they are not inherently problematic; instead, they are vital forces that contribute to the richness of life. Healthy Fire means we may encounter emotional stimuli (subtle or not) that throw us in one direction or another, but we're ultimately able to come back to a stable presence fairly easily.

In the Chinese medicine view of the body-mind, the Fire element organs of the Heart and Pericardium help us restore order and return to connection and a sense of meaning after a traumatic experience. As the master regulator and the empress of the body and mind, the Heart's steady and consistent beat tells the entire system that the threat has passed and it's safe to once again be with others, experience joy, and rest in equanimity. The Pericardium acts as an energetic buffer to protect the Heart physically but also psychologically. Energetically it provides a guarded barrier between our sensitive feelings and vulnerabilities and the outside world, and it holds the job of opening and closing, allowing people in at times that are nourishing and maintaining boundaries at other times. In particular, after a stressful event, it helps us restore social engagement and human connection. When we're closed down and not open to connecting with others—or when we're too open and easily betrayed or wounded—our Fire element has become imbalanced.

If we don't have space and time to return to balance after a stressful event, or we continue to be under regular traumatic threat, these organs can't do their regulatory work, and we may have trouble balancing the Fire element and settling the Heart-Mind. Because the domain of the Fire element is relationships, we may find it difficult to engage, feel safe, or develop intimacy with others. Another possibility is that we're overtaken by a kind of unrooted "joy" or mania, a sort of disembodied excitability that inhibits our ability to be present and connect meaningfully. During shock or a traumatic experience of any kind, your body's natural survival response causes you to orient toward external threats or danger. In extreme cases, we say the mind "leaves" the body, causing dissociation or a profound numbing or freezing. From the perspective of TCM, if a person is not able to restore coherence and instead finds themselves hypervigilant, always on edge, or swinging between depressive and anxious states, this is an indication that the Heart-Mind has scattered. This can happen with a small shock, such as a simple fender bender, or a severer event that leaves a more lasting imprint. In Chinese medicine, we call this a Shen or spirit disturbance. In such a case, we may need to do deliberate work to bring the spirit back home to the body.

The question when healing this aspect of the Fire element is "How can I settle my Heart-Mind and reconnect to my inner guidance and inner ground?" This is not always easy work and may, at times, require therapeutic support from skilled helpers and healers of all kinds. However, there are also many ways you can heal disconnection on your own, in your community, or with your loved ones. The suggestions and practices at the end of this and the next chapter will help you regain balance and kindle the steady glow of your Heart-Mind.

Habits for Disconnection

> Focus on reestablishing presence in your body. Access to our inner world begins with the strengthening and stabilizing forces of Qi and Jing (touched on in Part One) primarily held in our lower abdomen. We explore this energetic area, where your original life forces are stored—called the Field of Elixir—in chapter 11. Choose a few tasks you do every day—like standing in line or waiting at a red light—or choose a few specific times of day. At that moment, practice yoking to the present moment by bringing your awareness into your lower abdomen and simply noticing your breath and any sensations in your body. You can also nonjudgmentally observe if there are any feelings or moods arising. Remember, body-based, present-moment awareness is not intellectual or theoretical. If you get stuck in a narrative, return to the sensations in your body that are attached to your thinking, memories, and beliefs.

> Keep your eyes open. If you feel like your Heart-Mind has absorbed a shock and you are still caught in a trauma response, softly maintain some of your attention on the outer world during your yoga or meditation practice, while still attending to your internal felt sense. This will allow you to hear the messages of your body while remaining connected to your environment, teaching your

Heart-Mind that the stressor has passed and it's safe to settle in the present moment.

› Work with the pace of your practice. When practicing yoga or other forms of mindful movement, notice the pace at which you're practicing. At first, your body-mind may need faster movement, especially if you're feeling overly anxious or agitated. If that's the case, you might start your yoga practice with a few Sun Salutations or a short flow. However, over time slowing down is essential in trauma recovery. Stressful events often happen quickly, and that speed gets trapped inside you, which overwhelms your nervous system and Heart-Mind. If you usually move quickly, practice slowing the rhythm of your movement and breath during your practice, and aim to listen to the subtler sensations in your body.

THE HEART'S TRUTH

The sensory organ linked to the Fire element is the tongue. In Chinese medicine, we say the Heart "opens to the tongue," meaning our speech is a direct reflection of what lies in our Heart-Mind. The Fire element is also closely tied to the quality of our relationships, which depend on heartfelt communication. When you have a healthy Fire element, the speech conveyed via your tongue is internally rooted in your Heart.

Mindful Meditation Dyad Practice

For this exercise, you'll need a partner. Sit across from one another in comfortable meditation postures. In this practice, you'll take turns speaking your experience out loud during meditation. Whenever I offer this practice in the longer retreats I teach, students are surprised to discover how much they learn from and enjoy it after they overcome their initial resistance toward being so open and vulnerable with their partner. If you notice resistance arising within you, acknowledge it and give yourself some care, but I still encourage you to try the practice even if you're hesitant.

Begin by deciding who will be the questioner and who will be the responder. Once you have chosen, you can set a timer for 7 minutes to begin. Take your seats and feel your breath and body. Once you are present, the questioner asks, "How is it now?" The responder remains in meditation and replies with whatever they are experiencing in their body at that moment—for instance, "I'm feeling some heat in my hands," or "I'm feeling my chest moving with my breath." Both of you keep your attention gently focused on your experience by feeling sensations in your body. You may notice that new feelings, thoughts, or sensations arise due to the presence of someone else. That's okay. Stay aware of your own body and observe how sensations come and go.

As you practice, the questioner continues to repeat the same question: "How is it now?" Your pacing can vary, but allow your partner enough space to check in and be present. There is no rush in this practice. Simply be in the moment, witnessing. When the timer goes off, say thank you to your partner, switch roles, and go again. Avoid a lot of chatting about what you discovered between turns. Rather, stay in a meditative attitude until both of you have completed each role.

PRACTICES FOR BALANCE

Practices that support blood circulation, cultivate joy, and build a little heat in the body while maintaining ease and grounding support our Fire element. When working with Fire, we often need a mix of dynamic and recuperative practices to balance Fire and Water. Try a hybrid practice that includes both Yang-style and Yin-style practices to create harmony. Movements that target the structures around the heart, upper back, diaphragm, arms, and chest—where the Fire element meridians lie—are also helpful. In particular, supported backbends and arm balances harmonize the movement of Qi through the Fire element subtle body channels. If you experience anxiety, insomnia, restlessness, or a feeling of heat in your body, forward bends will help to counteract Fire and support introspection and cooling. Trauma-sensitive practices emphasizing self-care and kindness are also crucial when healing the Fire element.

Balasana (Child's Pose) with Courtyard of Spirit

———

Balasana is great for the Fire element because it is cooling and calming. In this particular variation, we'll include a few acupressure points to calm your mind and spirit.

To begin, come onto your mat and sit back on your heels, with your feet together and your knees apart. Keeping your hips close to your heels, lean forward and bring your head toward the floor. If your head doesn't reach the floor, place a soft support under it. If you experience discomfort in your ankles, knees, or hips, place padding under or around them until you're at ease. If you're feeling particularly fatigued and would like to use the pose as a restorative tonic, use bolsters and blankets for complete support until you don't feel any pressure or stretch. That version is particularly helpful to release your lower back and create a sense of safety and calm. You can place your arms and hands out in front of you or beside you, whichever is comfortable for you.

As you settle, soften your inner groin and allow the weight of your body to sink. Take a few deep breaths and aim to relax tension in and around your hips and belly. Soften your face, relax your jaw, and drop into the present moment. Feel your breath and body.

After a few breath cycles, bring your awareness to your midline—in the area from between your eyebrows to just beyond your hairline. A number of marma and acupoints that help to calm the mind and spirit are located here. You may already notice gentle pressure on these points as you bow your head onto your yoga mat or prop. In the area between your eyebrows is a point called Hall of Impressions (Yin Tang), which we discussed in Chapter 5. Just beyond your hairline is another point called Courtyard of Spirit (*Shen Ting*), which is very close to the marma point *Kapala*, meaning ruler of time. Ayurvedic physician Vasant Lad says this point is for those who often feel rushed and "bound by time." Along with calming the Heart-Mind, the Courtyard of Spirit point also clears pathogenic Wind, which can rise upward, causing a scattered mind, anxiety, or insomnia. The meridian on which this point lies—the Du, or Governing Vessel—is particularly important because of its relationship to the brain and the way in which it connects the brain and Heart. For the next few minutes, as you rest in Balasana, gently rock your head back and forth and up and down to massage these points.

When you feel ready, you can release, lift up, and place your knees together.

Breathing Air into Fire with Salamba Matsyasana (Supported Fish Pose)

Many people experience weakness or collapse in and around the area of the lungs and diaphragm. But Fire needs to breathe! Just as we blow a little air on kindling to encourage a flame, our Fire element needs air. Freedom in breathing supports the circulation of Qi or Prana and, therefore, good Fire element health. Lastly, the membranes of the physical heart and pericardium connect to the fascia of the diaphragm, so easy breathing contributes to healthy blood flow in the heart.

This movement, called Matsyasana, helps to open the lungs and chest and lengthens the front body, inviting more space and ease when breathing. It also supports good cervical curvature, which helps if you have chronically held tension in and around your upper back, shoulders, and neck. In this practice, we will do a supported variation. Many students need to start practicing this pose with a thinner prop and work toward more height over time. We'll ease into it here by using a rolled blanket.

Start by placing a firm blanket roll on your mat, parallel to the front edge of the mat. Sit in front of the blanket roll with your legs bent and feet on the floor. Lean back onto the blanket and rest your shoulder blades directly on the roll. Make sure that the lower borders of your shoulder blades are fixed to the prop, effectively creating a slight downward drag on your shoulders. Arch your neck so your head rests on the floor. If this causes too much neck compression or discomfort, you can place an additional thin blanket underneath your head.

In the final position, the blanket roll underneath you will create a spreading effect in your intercostal muscles, gently opening your chest and ribs. Relax and invite your body to release into the blanket. Reach your arms overhead, clasp your elbows, and reach your elbows and arms back toward the floor behind you. If you don't have the range in your shoulders for that movement, simply extend your arms out to the sides at whatever angle feels best. Stay in the pose for 1 to 3 minutes, breathing steadily and softly. To release, bring your arms down beside you, press firmly into your elbows and forearms, inhale, and lift straight up through the center.

Ganesha Mudra

This mudra (hand gesture) is named after the elephant-headed deity Lord Ganesha, the remover of obstacles. Ganesha is a powerful and compassionate guardian—he protects the innocent. Invoking the power of Ganesha helps support strong discriminating boundaries, especially when we feel we have been violated or need some extra steadiness and courage after a shock.

When you are practicing meditation, you can use the Ganesha Mudra or visualize Ganesha at the doorway to your inner world to remember an internal sense of support and bolster your inner resolve and strength.

To begin, sit in a comfortable meditation posture. Keep your spine upright and your belly and breath soft. Begin by bringing your hands into a prayer position. Then swivel one palm so it is facing out and the other so it is facing toward the body, with your fingers pointing toward the opposite elbow. Now curl your fingers in and interlock or clasp them. The palms should not touch each other. Press your fingers firmly against each other and try to

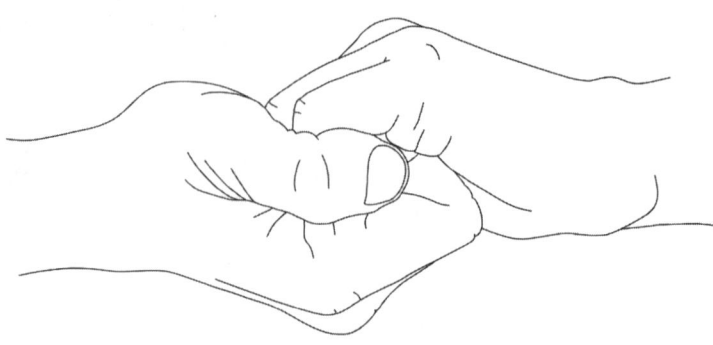

pull them apart gently. This creates a firm connection in the mudra. Take a few soft, deep breaths and feel the confidence this mudra elicits.

Shaking Practice

Have you ever seen an animal shake its body after a threat or stressful experience? Shaking is a powerful somatic practice we can use to balance our Fire element, release tension, connect with the body, process traumatic stress, and reset the nervous system.

Choose a quiet, private place where you feel comfortable and safe. You can do this practice standing up, as described here, or you can do a similar practice seated or lying down. Start by grounding. Stand with your feet hip-width apart, knees slightly bent, and arms relaxed by your sides. Take a few deep breaths, inhaling through your nose and sighing out through your mouth. Begin by gently bouncing on your feet. Let the movement travel upward through your body. Let your body go and give yourself over to the movement. Now begin to amplify your shaking. Shake your legs, hips, torso, arms, and head as it feels right for you. Let go of any need to control the movement. If it feels natural, add sounds like sighing, humming, or even vocal expressions to release tension. Stay present; notice where your body feels tight or heavy. Focus on shaking those areas. Let emotions, memories, or sensations arise without judgment. Shake for 30 seconds to 2 minutes.

To complete your practice, gradually reduce the intensity of your shaking, letting your movements become smaller and slower until you come to stillness. Stand or sit quietly for a few minutes. Place your hands over your heart or belly and simply notice any sensations, thoughts, or feelings.

Checking in with the Pulse of Your Heart with Great Gateway

Find a comfortable meditation posture; you can sit or lie down. Relax your body, soften or close your eyes, and tune in. Begin by following a few cycles of your breath. Aim to settle your thoughts and relax into your body. Once you feel quiet, place your hand on your chest a little left of center. Sense your physical heart just beneath your rib cage. Observe the beating of this powerful organ and the pulse of blood throughout your body. If you're having difficulty feeling your pulse, you can place your fingers on your neck at your carotid artery for a few moments.

Next, slide your hand down to rest just below your sternocostal angle, which is on the midline of your body just below the ribs. This is where an acupoint called Great Gateway (*Ju Que*) lies. This subtle energetic area is where the Qi of your Heart organ gathers. In my acupuncture practice, I use it in cases of overexcitability or depression. We can tap into its subtle power here with our mindful awareness. As you rest your hand on this area, sense again the pulsatory movement of blood.

After a few minutes of sensing this rhythm, release your hands and feel the sensation directly. Relax and sink into the feeling of your heart's constant and continual beat. Imagine your energetic Heart inside you— the empress that holds your inner truth. Simply attend to this area with presence and be open to any messages from within. Stay with this practice for 10 to 15 minutes.

This chapter explored how we can become disconnected from our higher truth when the Fire element is imbalanced and some habits and methods to harmonize Fire. In the next chapter, we'll move on to its subtle aspects, including emotional and spiritual imbalance and associated practices.

NINE

EMPTY MIND, OPEN HEART

To find the soul one must step back from the surface, (go) deep within, and enter, enter . . . and then there is something warm, tranquil, rich, very still, and very full, like a sweetness . . .
—MIRRA ALFASSA

Since the beginning of time, humans have gathered around bonfires under the fiery light of stars to share stories, songs, and sorrow. Like the bonfire, when our Fire element is healthy, it invites us into inclusive communion with others and ourselves. It empowers us to be vulnerable, to step into the circle, and to share ourselves fully. It welcomes us to see and experience our connection with the whole and remember the divine light inside. As the theologian Elizabeth A. Johnson says, "For all our distinctiveness, human beings are modes of being of the universe. Woven into our lives is the very fire from the stars and genes from the sea creatures, and everyone, utterly everyone, is kin in the radiant tapestry of being. This relationship is not external or extrinsic to who we are but wells up as the defining truth from our deepest being"[26] Healthy Fire teaches us how to be in clear relationship with ourselves and others, to love this world passionately and with abandon, and to celebrate it with all our hearts.

The emotion we associate most often with Fire is usually called joy or overexcitement. It can also include a certain kind of anxiety, agitation, or extreme mania that feels hot and fast. When in balance, it's the feeling of being alive and open, and there's a fresh sense of happiness that remains anchored to a sense of self. It's interesting that, in the Chinese classics, both characters used to refer to this emotion indicate music. Joy is what brings us together to sing, dance, and celebrate. Remembering that the movement of Fire is up and out like a growing flame, we can see how the outward movement of joy is Fire's emotion. Joy and excitement expand and spread and, when out of balance, can cause our Qi and spirit to scatter like embers blowing in the wind.

When first examining the Five Element model, it's easy to think that Fire gets the good emotion, joy, while all the other elements are stuck with the so-called negative ones, like anger or grief. But the truth is every emotion is simply moving energy. Each has its time and can be either in or out of balance. Our culture leans toward believing we need to be joyful all the time, but just as we can't live in summer all year round, we can't be joyous all the time either. The right amount of each emotion at the right time keeps us healthy and is, of course, a part of life.

Even with joy, things can get out of balance. Have you ever been so ecstatic that you almost felt your heart skip a beat or you wanted to just jump for joy? Think of a child who has had a little too much sugar or someone in your life who laughs too much or is always on the lookout for more excitement. When our Fire element is in excess, we move too far outside ourselves, and everything speeds up. We may try to avoid anything that brings the mood "down" and instead continually seek out more fun. While there's nothing wrong with entertainment and play, trying to be joyful all the time can be tiring. When I have a patient like this, I usually identify Heat in their body-mind in the form of rapid or excessive communication and faster movement. Sometimes folks with this excess will have poor boundaries in their relationships, and in the extreme, they may display signs of manic behavior.

On the other hand, too little of this powerful emotion, and we may feel flat and joyless. After all, the Fire element is the spark of life! Because the outward movement of Fire is so important in maintaining relationships, when our Fire element is deficient, we might not have the desire or vitality for connection with others and feel lonely much of the time. Without Fire, we also lack the ability to experience true intimacy with ourselves and others. This can show up as a disconnection from a sense of self or as an inability to bond emotionally or physically. Without a connection to our inner joy, we may fall head over heels in love too quickly or end up in relationships that take advantage of our vulnerability and need for closeness. Either way, when this emotion is imbalanced, we lose contact with a deeper aspect of ourselves.

The Chinese classics tell us joy injures the Heart. The key to working with this emotion is finding the right amount of Fire and experiencing happiness in a mindful way. The true nature of our empress, the Heart, is not anxious or excitable. Instead, the Heart is an empty space that can hold all things. Just like a flower stays rooted as it blooms, joy blossoms into presence and warmth when we stay connected to ourselves internally. When we embody this, we not only balance joy, we also transform it into Fire's higher vibration, a sense of inner guidance, which balances both awareness and care (a subject we'll explore in the next two sections).

THE SPIRIT OF FIRE

Out of all the types of consciousness outlined in TCM, the spirit of our Heart and Fire element, the Shen, is the only one actually translated as "spirit" or "consciousness." The term *Shen* is unique in that it refers not only to the spirit that resides in the Heart but also to all the states of consciousness that are associated with the elements and organs.

According to Daoist thought, the key to understanding the Shen of the Heart, and the psychospiritual qualities of the Fire element in general, is in understanding how the clarity of the mind and the sensitive, loving heart are deeply intermingled and ultimately inseparable. In light of this, I often refer to the Heart and the Shen as the Heart-Mind, because it's responsible for feeling *and* thought. Essentially, the Shen is our inner heartfelt knowing and truth. If we nurture a spiritual outlook and develop greater heart-centered wakefulness, the Shen can act as an inner guiding light throughout our lives.

This is similar to yoga and Buddhism where the mind has multiple interdependent functions. The first domain of mind is more linear; it looks to the world and gives things names and attributes. We identify and separate things we experience through our senses in order to understand them. For instance, the mind looks at the sky and identifies a "cloud." From there, the mind attaches any number of preferences, opinions, and memories to the cloud. As the mind separates the cloud and turns it into an object, it loses the view that this cloud is part of a much larger tapestry of life; it significantly reduces it to a single "thing." This cloud is essential to the whole, of course. It was once the rain, the rain was once the earth, the earth was once our bodies, and so on.

The second part of our mind is *citta*, which is often translated as heart. Citta is sometimes used to refer to thought itself, but it's also the unwavering consciousness beneath thought. It is our innermost being. Citta receives everything, is informed by our conditioning, and creates our sense of self. Most often, citta is caught in a never-ending cycle of reactions. However, when it is able to let go of these projections, it realizes its own profound, open, and unshakable nature, a nature that goes way beyond preference or thought (unconditional heart-mind, called *cit*, is equal to *purusha*, or our "inner light of awareness"). As you can see, this realm of the Heart-Mind has the capacity for cognition as well as open, loving awareness. The foremost aim of yoga is a refinement of citta, which culminates in a higher state of inner awareness. Later in this chapter, we'll explore practices to guide the part of the mind that rationalizes and divides into a more receptive, open, and clarified citta as a way to support Shen.

In TCM, Shen is one of the revered Three Treasures (Jing, Qi, and Shen), which we touched on in Part One. The Shen is the most refined substance of the three; assessing it gives me an indication of my patient's mental, spiritual, and emotional health. Shen, in particular, relies on the nourishment of healthy Blood to rest and Qi and Jing for energy and substance. The health of those substances is nourished through all the primary ways we take care of ourselves—a healthy diet, good sleep, the right amount of exercise, and so forth. If Qi and Jing are strong, our Shen and mental health will generally be stable. If Qi and Jing are deficient, our Shen will suffer, and we'll feel unsettled, anxious, or depressed. The physician Zhang Jie Bin emphasizes the close relationship between the Three Treasures in his historic medical text, the *Lei Jing*: "If the Jing is strong, Qi flourishes; if Qi flourishes, the Shen is whole."[27]

The spark of Shen lands inside each of us at conception. You see it in a baby's eyes with the first hints of awareness as that little being begins to absorb the outer world. As we grow, our Shen contributes to clarity of thought, restful sleep, and emotional balance. Remember, the term *Shen* represents the consciousness and faculties of both the mind and the energetic Heart. It's associated with thinking, the senses, memory, feeling, insight, and ideas. It also determines how we connect with ourselves and each other. Through these responsibilities, the Shen plays a very important role in determining our overall psychological, emotional, and even spiritual health. For example, without the inner guidance of the Shen and Heart-Mind, a person may lack refined insight and presence. They may be more negatively affected by emotional upheaval or, as we'll see later in this chapter, more likely to use spirituality to bypass difficult or unsavory aspects of self.

It's interesting to note that the Heart is often depicted as an empty space in Eastern systems. For instance, the Chinese character for *Heart* shows an empty vessel, along with illustrating the physical structures of the organ. This empty center highlights the ability of our Shen spirit to allow and accept all things with love. Whether it's an interpersonal challenge at work, the sorrow of a world gone mad, a brilliant ocean view, or the elation of true love, a fully integrated and balanced Heart-Mind can hold what Daoists call the "ten thousand things." The Buddhist teacher Ajahn Chah highlights the capacity of the awakened and resourced Heart-Mind this way:

> Try to be mindful, and let things take their natural course. Then your mind will become still in any surroundings, like a clear forest pool. All kinds of wonderful, rare animals will come to drink at the pool, and you will clearly see the nature of all things. You will see many strange and wonderful things come and go, but you will be still. This is the happiness of the Buddha.[28]

Consciousness or awareness, the Shen, resides in the empty space of the Heart. It has the capacity to bear with ease all that passes through it.

A SPACE TO HOLD ALL THINGS

Unfortunately, many people have lost contact with the true nature of their Heart, their bright-yet-spacious and empty inner light. Our modern culture assaults and desensitizes this vulnerable center in many ways. Within a capitalist and often extremely competitive environment, it's not always easy to stay in touch with and support the qualities of a healthy and integrated Heart-Mind. Rather than turn inward, the current culture encourages us to sacrifice a deeper, heart-centered knowing and use only our minds in search of the latest shiny thing. For hundreds of years, the colonial project has valued the accrual of wealth and power over almost everything else, including human life and the sanctity of the planet. It's like being mesmerized by an action-packed movie or lulled to sleep by a powerful drug. Looking outside ourselves, we follow the pull of the mind rather than listen to the murmurings of the Heart.

When we value "me" and "mine" over care for and connection to our shared humanity, the mind has split from the Heart and, for the most part, acts separately from it. The undeveloped mind, when separated in this way, understands only by thinking and seeing the world through its own views and opinions. Because the nature of the mind on its own is generally to avoid pain and seek pleasure, it operates without much care for the larger web of life. We forget that there is no first prize at the end of the line. In this scenario, the mind lacks the softening perspective of the Heart and is continually caught in habitual reactions to emotion and thought.

This all sounds pretty dire, but there is a way to bring Heart and Mind back together. When we accomplish this, we're able to be with each brilliant thing without desire for some fantasyland. In fact, when we remember to look inward, we discover the Heart and Mind were connected all along. The Zen master Huang Po describes it this way:

> Your true nature is something never lost to you even in moments of delusion, nor is it gained at the moment of enlightenment. . . .

It is all-pervading, spotless beauty; it is the self-existent and un-created Absolute.[29]

The true nature of your Heart-Mind is sometimes called your "original luminous brilliance." It remains ever-present and is always inside you. The human mind holds immense possibilities, but it can easily be manipulated and swayed. The good news is that at any time, we can access the luminous brilliance that is the true nature of an integrated Heart-Mind—for guidance, connection, insight, and spacious support.

The Fire element and the powerful transformative force of the Heart-Mind can be cultivated and stoked through awareness practices. However, the penetrating clarity of awareness can be like fire; if not moderated, it will be out of balance and can even become destructive. This is why methods that cultivate awareness also require a balancing of techniques that emphasize care. Practices that build kindness toward ourselves and others can help balance and temper the more exacting practices that require precise and concentrated awareness. Including a heart-centered approach in our spiritual practice can help us relate to whatever experiences arise with greater understanding and acceptance. Without this balance of clarity *and* compassion, we risk becoming unhinged in a variety of ways, allowing the mind free rein without loving guidance.

In my classes, I use the classical analogy of a beautiful bird to describe these two essential parts of practice. There is the wing of mindfulness and the wing of compassionate acceptance. Each wing is necessary and supports the other. Mindfulness helps us see what is here, be it heartbreak, abandonment, or trepidation; compassion and kindness allow us to meet it with tenderness. For example, when we are mindful of being anxious, we can become aware of our sweaty palms, our racing thoughts, or our stilted breath. We may feel frozen or compelled to act out. Our wing of compassion gives us the ability to soften around the experience and relate to it in a sympathetic way; this helps us be with what is here even if we want to run away or wish it would change or end.

If we learn only to clarify the mind and pay attention, our focus will become sharp and clear, but we won't necessarily be able to meet whatever we find skillfully. We risk becoming cold and detached or caving to judgment and aversion. Heart practices keep us tethered; they help us see what is there with a quality of warmth and loving-kindness.

Unfortunately, there are many examples of spiritual teachers who have attained high levels of awareness in the mind without the same level of development in their Hearts. Without a grounding in kindness and good emotional intelligence, a practitioner risks becoming disconnected, self-centered, or (at the very worst) harmful to others. I first learned the term *spiritual bypassing* from the gifted psychologist John Welwood, with whom I had the privilege of practicing and studying on a number of occasions. Spiritual bypassing describes how some modern spiritual practitioners try to skip important stages of psychological development or uneasy emotional material prematurely. When a person spiritually bypasses, they misuse spiritual teachings and practices to reinforce unhealthy ways of being and relating. While the full scope of this concept is beyond the range of our discussion, the essence of it speaks perfectly to what we're exploring. The human experience is messy, and pretending we're more "spiritual" than human seems to be an easy way out. However, when we use our practices to avoid the unsavory and inflate our sense of specialness rather than face what is difficult or connect with our Hearts' knowing, we're most likely bypassing. Even if we try to avoid it, our shadow material doesn't just go away; it still informs our understanding and ability to progress on the path.

Another example of this disconnect between Mind and Heart is how we might use our practice as just another tool in a never-ending self-improvement project. We may initially come to yoga or meditation because it helps us feel more at ease or content, but eventually the mind can turn toward wanting to be better or feeling inadequate. Our habits of self-loathing and not-enoughness are so powerful that breaking them requires a conscious and active effort. Fortunately, the all-knowing and supportive empress of our Heart-Mind offers us the perfect antidote to self-criticism. We don't need to change the aspects of ourselves that don't neatly conform to our ideal. Rather, we can get to know and come to understand all the places within and meet them with kindness, regardless of their flavor.

Chinese medicine and Daoism teach us that we can't rigidly follow the desires of the imagined self if we're to maintain harmony and flow. Being in the Dao is a delicate dance, one in which we must accept all aspects of our experience. I like to imagine following my path as a practice of lightly touching things with an open hand. When we hold to things too tightly, the Heart-Mind clamps down and is restricted from expressing its natural state, which is to bloom, open, and connect with clarity and care. The more we try to maintain control, the more we lack presence. When we follow the Dao with a sense of openness, we allow things to be the way they are, and we surrender to the intuitive knowing of our Heart, which includes both awareness and love.

Our practice of joining Heart and Mind begins with our own broken selves—our wounds, fears, and numbness—but we soon discover that this path of Heart is wide. It has the potential to hold not only our own grief, apathy, disconnection, and rage but also the pains of the whole living world. The Buddhist teacher Pema Chödrön says it this way:

> On the journey of the warrior-bodhisattva, the path goes down, not up, as if the mountain pointed toward the earth instead of the sky. Instead of transcending the suffering of all creatures, we move toward turbulence and doubt however we can. We explore the reality and unpredictability of insecurity and pain, and we try not to push it away. If it takes years, if it takes lifetimes, we let it be as it is. At our own pace, without speed or aggression, we move down and down and down. With us move millions of others, our companions in awakening from fear. At the bottom we discover water, the healing water of bodhichitta. Bodichitta is our heart, our wounded, softened heart. Right down there in the thick of things, we discover the love that will not die. This love is bodhichitta. It is gentle and warm; it is clear and sharp; it is open and spacious. The awakened heart of bodhichitta is the basic goodness of all beings.[30]

When grounded in the Heart, we are influenced to do no harm and direct our fiery passions for the good of all beings.

Most practitioners experience feelings of care in the Heart and clarity in the mind as two separate phenomena. But remember, in Daoist, yogic, and Buddhist systems, the word for Heart and Mind is the same. So when you're practicing mindfulness, you could say you're practicing heart-fullness too! As we explore the nature of the Heart-Mind with the practices that follow, you may discover your feelings and thoughts are in direct relationship with one another. Thoughts feed emotion, and emotion triggers thought. In light of this, we'll explore how we might hold both struggle and joy with a practice of mindfulness along with *maitri*, a practice focused on loving-kindness.

HEALING THE FIRE ELEMENT

> Practice holding inner presence and open, joyful connection at the same time. Next time you're in a social setting, try to embody both engagement with others and connection to your innermost self. Can you stay connected internally while moving outward? To connect with others and develop healthy relationships, we need to be okay with the Fire energy of excitement, which is very close to the feeling of anxiety. What's it like to be okay with some fire-like feelings? Can you stay open (with safe boundaries) even when you have a history of being hurt or experiencing pain? Can you allow and accept the wounded places within without letting them shut you down and close you off? To maintain Fire element balance, the more joy you radiate outward, the more bonding to your inner truth and root you need.

> Infuse your practice and life with the flavor of acceptance. What would it be like to loosen the reins of control a little? This isn't about apathy or not caring. In fact, it's the opposite. Letting go of the things that don't matter helps us open to what does. Next time you're on your yoga mat or meditation cushion, focus on bringing an attitude of relaxation and ease into every movement and breath. Emphasize releasing clinging, fixing, and adjusting a bit more. In your daily activities, rather than adding more to-do lists, self-judgments, and expectations, can you bring more lightness of spirit, humor, or a sense of unity to your life? The more often you

can let things be, the more directly you'll be able to experience the clarity, space, and presence of your Heart-Mind.

> Practice balancing your Mind and Heart. Next time you sit down to meditate, see if you can feel the warmth of your own Heart. Can you also feel the clarity of your mind and thoughts? First, focus on these two separately and then bring them together. Is one stronger for you than the other? What is it like to work with both aspects simultaneously?

Mindfulness with an Open Heart-Mind

Find a comfortable posture, whether sitting or lying down. Set your timer for 15 minutes. Gently close your eyes and take a few deep, calming breaths. Start by spending a few minutes simply feeling your body and breath.

Next, shift your attention to your Heart-Mind. Notice any emotions or thoughts that arise. These thoughts may be about the past, the future, or the present moment. Observe them without judgment. As you continue to meditate, imagine your Heart-Mind as a clear blue sky. Thoughts are like clouds passing through this sky. Throughout this meditation, aim to see your thoughts clearly with an attitude of kindness. Whenever you notice your attention wandering, come back to your breath and this spacious, open sky. As each thought arises, observe any feelings or sensations that accompany it. Simply acknowledge whatever arises and let it go, allowing it to drift away like a cloud.

As you settle, notice any patterns or tendencies in your thinking. Are your thoughts predominantly positive or negative? Are they focused on a specific topic? Observe these patterns without getting caught up in them. Approach every thought with a spacious mind and a caring Heart.

Recall something in your life that has been a positive influence on you. This may be a person like a mentor, a place you enjoy visiting, or even a pet. Feel the impact of having this source of support. As you consider this positive force, notice any thoughts or feelings that arise in the open sky of your awareness. You might also notice any sensations in your body. Once again, allow thoughts to come and go without getting enmeshed in them.

Next, bring to mind something that is a source of struggle or suffering. Don't dive directly into the most difficult situation, but do stay present with something that causes you some kind of pain. Once again observe any thoughts, feelings, or sensations that present themselves. As they arise, allow them to pass through without trying to fix, figure out, or change anything. Approach what you discover with both a clear mind and an open Heart.

Now allow both situations to be present simultaneously. Stay with your breath and notice what it's like to hold both situations with openness and care in the vast sky of your Heart-Mind. Remember that the Heart-Mind has the capacity for both clear perception and loving care. As you rest in this space, know that an available Heart-Mind can hold your joys and sorrows equally. As you complete your meditation, take a moment to observe the state of your mind now. How has your mental state changed?

THE DIVINE ABIDINGS

In Buddhism and yoga, the four heavenly abodes, or divine abidings (*brahma viharas*) are a set of inner attitudes that are essential to cultivate in order to support the true nature of the Heart-Mind. These states of being are foundational to the spiritual path. They balance and soften the sharp and rigorous qualities of mindfulness and help us relate to our human experience with skill and presence. As we develop these qualities, they help us have a warmhearted attitude toward ourselves and all living beings. They are maitri (loving-kindness), karuna (compassion), *mudita* (sympathetic joy), and *upeksha* (equanimity). In this practice, we'll explore maitri.

One of the most common ways of practicing maitri is by internally reciting phrases of kindness first toward ourselves, then to those we don't know, those with whom we have difficulty, and finally to all beings. The simplicity of this practice allows us to use it almost anywhere and anytime. You can try it when you're out in the world or in seated meditation. As you do this, you're supporting your Fire element, Shen, and Heart-Mind. Plus, you're actually creating new neural pathways that encourage greater acceptance, love, and happiness.

Remember, maitri is a *purification* practice; as you aim to open your Heart, you may encounter all that stands in the way! Sometimes you may find it almost impossible to send love to yourself and others, at other times you'll find the practice uplifting and joyful. That's perfectly normal. Just as we saw in Chapter 6, many hindrances can pop up during practice that can lead us away from presence. The same is true for developing the Heart. When we come to our practice, we bring not only the nice, loving, and content version of ourselves; we also bring the neurotic, lazy, controlling, and judgmental facets of our psyche. Encountering this reality can be a bit shocking. All of it is an essential step in the process. We must first discover how we shut down and turn away from love if we ever want to more fully open and accept it into our being.

As you repeat the phrases toward yourself and others, notice the way your heart contracts and expands in relation to your intention. Remember, this style of practice systematically uproots the inner narrative that persistently speaks and feels fear and separation. The transformation that is possible through dedicated practice has the potential to soften your heart and open you to the love that is accessible in every moment.

Loving-Kindness Practice

Maitri, or loving-kindness, is the foundational practice on which the other three divine abodes rest. It encompasses a boundless and unconditional love for all beings. Maitri arises out of a heartfelt desire for others' happiness and involves wishing well-being and peace for oneself and others without discrimination or attachment.

To begin, try repeating one of the following phrases to yourself when you notice self-judgment cropping up or during a particular time every day (for example, before you fall asleep every night or at the end of your yoga practice). Feel free to alter the phrases so you feel a connection to the words. After all, the practice is to strengthen the capacity of *your*

Heart; it's not so much about affecting the other person as it is about changing your relationship to care. Try these phrases to begin:

> May I be well in body, mind, and spirit.
> May I be at peace internally and externally.
> May I feel connected, supported, and loved.
> May I be healthy, strong, and free.

As you practice, reflect: How does it feel? Allow whatever you experience to be present without judgment. As your practice strengthens, you can try directing your phrases first toward a loved one, then a neutral person, then a person with whom you have difficulty, and finally, all beings everywhere; for example, "May *you* be well in body, spirit, and mind."

As you practice, if you feel blocked in any way toward a person or situation, remember that developing care can help to clarify your aversion. Most likely, the person you are thinking of is also suffering on some level. What would it be like to recognize that they struggle too? This technique is not about masking important feelings or condoning bad behavior. It's about transforming your Heart so you can stay open even when you feel aversion or disagreement. This way, what was once confusing or destructive is now something more refined and healing.

We've explored how the Yang energy of the Fire element is expressed as resplendent maturation and expansion. All life thrives when imbued with this zest. When balanced, it provides ample joyous energy and supports access to our divine spirit. In the Five Element cycle, Fire's ashes create the Earth element. The transition from Fire to Earth is one of reestablishing balance and finding your ground. In our next section we'll investigate the season of centering and the many manifestations of the Earth element.

LATE SUMMER SEASON & EARTH ELEMENT

TEN

LATE SUMMER HARVEST & THE EARTH ELEMENT

What if we could fashion a restoration plan that grew from understanding multiple meanings of land? Land as sustainer. Land as identity. Land as grocery store and pharmacy. Land as connection to our ancestors. Land as moral obligation. Land as sacred. Land as self.[31]

—ROBIN WALL KIMMERER

Now, we enter the Earth phase of the Five Element cycle. Of course, earth is the name of our beautiful, diverse, and abundant home; the only planet we know of that can sustain human life. The Earth element is the rich soil we stand on that grows our food and the sweet nourishment we receive when we digest that food well. Earth nurtures life in all its natural manifestations—the dank marshes, great open plains, rich rolling hills, and verdant valleys. In Chinese medicine and Daoism, this element represents our regular rhythms and routines and all that cradles and grounds us. You can also see the Earth element as the hearth, the nurturing center of your home—a place of comfort, belonging, and sanctuary. Earth is one of the most material elements; in our bodies, it generally represents the physicality of our flesh. Quite literally, we come from earth through the food we eat, and one day we will return to earth's warm embrace. Through an act of transformation, this element builds the body and mind by receiving nutrients from organic matter

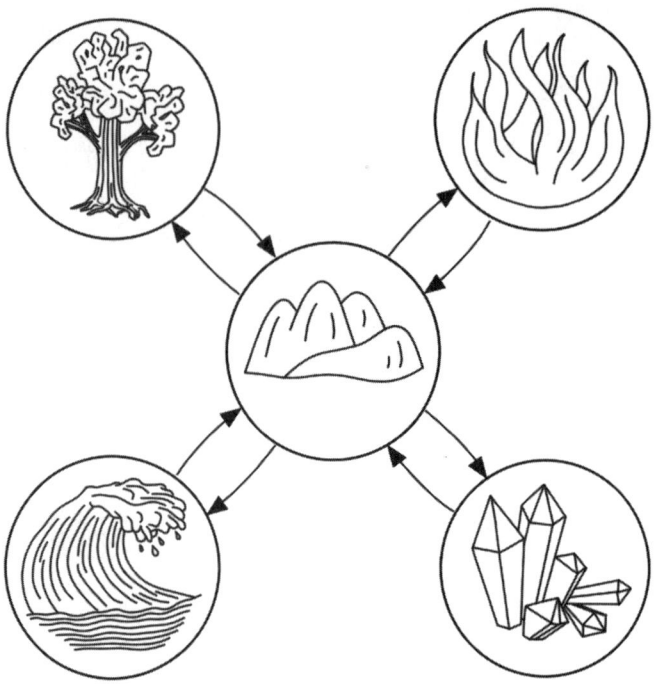

and assimilating them into sustenance and energy. On a psychospiritual level, the Earth element gives us a sense of center. It keeps us connected to our intentions and helps us transform our thoughts into something material.

In the Five Element cycle, Earth is a place of balance that occurs momentarily between each element and season. It acts as a kind of center point, a brief place of neutrality and equilibrium within the natural wheel of change. While the other elemental energies connect to movement (growth and decline, for example), we link the Earth element to stability and grounding. Our planet earth sustains us because it stays steady even while it constantly spins on its axis. As a center point, Earth supports all other elements with its ability to nurture, hold, and transform. It provides a grounded place for the growth of the Wood element's plants; the Fire element's molten center; the mountain peaks and precious minerals of the Metal element; and the rivers, creeks, and great oceans of the Water element. The earth is the symbolic mother in many cultures worldwide—from the ancient Greek Gaia to the numerous stories of the Earth Mother in First Nations and aboriginal teachings to Pachamama, the Incan fertility goddess. Interestingly, the words *matter* and *matrix* derive from the same etymological root, *mater*, meaning "mother." Our fertile Mother Earth gives us the energy, stability, comfort, and support to manifest material rewards like a gorgeous garden or meal, a complete manuscript or project, or a fulfilling relationship and family from our dedicated labor and intentions.

Along with its unique characteristic of representing the transition and balance point between each elemental state and season, the Earth element is commonly placed after Fire and before Metal. It's especially apparent during late summer, the transitional period of balance between Yang (spring and summer) and Yin (fall and winter). Late summer is considered a distinct season in Five Element theory. Although we don't formally recognize it in the West, we still experience this relatively short seasonal juncture. For those of us living in the north, it usually occurs sometime in the later stages of summer with the last slivers of warmth and runs until about the first frost of early autumn. Late summer signifies a moment in the natural cycle when things seem to stand still for just a moment. It is where the downward pull of gravity and entropy increases as upward-moving, active qualities lessen.

During late summer, there is a lowering of intensity—the angle of light in the sky changes, a mellow dusting of bronze blankets the landscape, and there's a feeling of peace and prosperity in nature. There may be more weeks of hot weather left, but there's also a hint of decay in the air. In late summer, I notice more amber and rust-colored leaves on the forest floor, and my body craves a bit more slowness. During this transitional phase, the fast pace of summer relaxes, and time seems to thicken. As the wild grasses and grains turn golden, nature beckons us to savor what has matured and soak in the warmth of summer's last light.

Throughout this time, the abundance of the natural world is on full display; after much preparation and devotion, fruits and vegetables hang heavy and ripe, ready for gathering and sharing. Blackberry picking becomes a delightful priority. My garden basket usually brims with late summer rose hips, tomatoes, and basil, and the squash grow at an extraordinary rate. Many of the plants I've tended throughout spring and summer slowly go to seed, carried by the wind. At the farmers market, the arrival of apples, corn, and the first sweet pumpkin is a sure sign of the change of seasons. In late summer, I love exploring the forest beyond my home and sustainably wildcrafting many medicinal botanicals, which will become medicines for use throughout the year. This is harvest season, when we can finally celebrate our bounty and gratitude for the plentiful gifts of the earth.

The qualities of harmony and fulfillment naturally arise at this time of year. Earth herself delivers endlessly during this season; she fills our bubbling pots and sweet-smelling pies with her gifts, and even after the harvest is complete, when the land seems still, she holds seeds just beneath the surface in a cocoon of nurturing soil. As any farmer will tell you, Earth element season is also a busy time that requires much intentional work. To enjoy all this abundance, one must give generously to the land in order to receive. When I consider the qualities of the Earth element, I think of my dear husband, a skilled carpenter and designer. He can't rush the process of creating architectural designs or crafting beautiful furniture from wood. Taking his time, he carefully tends to his art until, eventually, he's ready to share his creation with others. Those who harmonize with the richness of late summer know the power of working slowly and with thanks, honoring the offerings of the earth.

Many traditions throughout the world mark the beginning of the late summer harvest. It's a time to offer gratitude for earth's abundance to ensure a successful yield. The Celtic and pagan traditions begin with Lughnasadh, a harvest festival focused on the first fruits and grains of the season, and follow that up with the festival of Mabon, which celebrates the autumn equinox when day and night are equal. The early Christian name for this celebration was Lammas, meaning "loaf mass," where the Church blessed specific breads. Since this holiday centers around cutting grain, festivities focus on bread, the staff of life. Traditionally, agricultural communities would come together to share the first harvest, often baking bread from the newly harvested grain. Communal feasts and the sharing of food and drink marked these gatherings. The midautumn festival in Chinese culture is usually near the autumn equinox and also celebrates all that is ripe and abundant this time of year with special foods and the lighting of lanterns. This season is a chance to come together with friends and family, neighbors, and our larger community to rejoice in the fruition of all we have sewn (ideally with a warm cup of mulled cider and some good company).

Just as the compost heap creates dark, fertile soil from the organic matter we put in it, we feed our bodies and minds with the rich wealth earth gives us. This is the essence of the Earth element—what was once natural abundance is now transformed, digested, and assimilated into deep nourishment and satisfaction. However, the Earth element is not only about enjoyment and gratification. To find balance we must learn to embody reciprocity—to live in a sincere way that acknowledges this nourishment is conditional. This way we act with integrity, the virtue associated with Earth, only taking what we need and always giving back in a balanced way.

EARTH IMAGERY AND LANGUAGE

A home-cooked meal

Family

Pumpkin pie

Plump fruits

A warm embrace

A bountiful garden plot

A mud puddle

Late afternoon

A warm kitchen

A caretaker

A beautiful nest

A hardworking craftsperson

Lullabies

Breastfeeding

Farms, rice paddies, fruit orchards

A compost pile

ENERGETICS OF EARTH CHART

Season	Late summer
Yin organ	Spleen
Yang organ	Stomach
Tissue	Muscles
Sense organ	Mouth
Emotion	Worry
Direction	Center
Sound	Singing
Climatic influence	Dampness
Taste	Sweet
Color	Yellow

SEASONAL SELF-CARE FOR LATE SUMMER

The Earth element influences the transitional periods between each of the four seasons. As pivot points, these are important times to cultivate equilibrium. In particular, late summer is a great time to find your center and aim for balance in all endeavors. Time seems to slow down, and all activity should be easy. Here are a few general suggestions for harmonizing or rebalancing your lifestyle during the late summer harvest season or any transitional period between seasons.

> Now is a time to pause, to enjoy all you have grown, and to reestablish balance if you are out of harmony. Check in and ask yourself if your levels of activity and rest are balanced. Have you recently overindulged? What is your work-life balance like? How can you create more evenness in the months to come?
> Aim for the middle path in your plans, actions, thoughts, and words. This is not a time for extremes, so rather than doing too much or too little or reacting strongly to the events of your life, can you develop more equanimity?
> Easy-to-digest experiences are best now. Don't add too much complexity to your schedule. The Earth element thrives when you

"digest" experience, so don't rush through significant events and changes. Instead, process them through journaling, moments of self-reflection, or sharing with a supportive person.

> Use activities and practices that are grounding. Try slow-moving yoga and standing practices that emphasize connection to the earth. Refer to practices in the next two chapters for ideas.
> Spend more time with your community and with those you love. Try hosting a potluck or a community meal to encourage deeper roots of support, generosity, and caring within your chosen community.
> Find what nourishes you—physically, mentally, emotionally, energetically, spiritually—and then do it!

LATE SUMMER HARVEST KITCHEN MEDICINE

During late summer, many foods mature. As they ripen, they build sugar and become more digestible. It's time to bring people together to enjoy and give thanks, to harvest the earth's bounty before it rots and releases to the ground.

You may remember, the Earth element is also a crucial time of transformation and nourishment and is present between each season or element. This is akin to the Ayurvedic concept of *ritusandhi*—a transitional period between two seasons. You can use these suggestions to reestablish balance and support your digestive capacity in the interchange between any of the seasons. The focus for Earth element nutrition should be on preparing and consuming foods that are simple, centering, and grounding, with an emphasis on the natural mildly sweet flavor. The health of your digestive system and warding off the pathogen Dampness are also particularly important. You'll find a more in-depth discussion of this in Chapter 11. If it's late summer, place special attention on reducing the accumulation of Heat (pitta dosha in Ayurveda) and preparing for autumn. Use the following suggestions to maintain good health in the kitchen during Earth element time:

> Slowly add more cooked foods to your diet and reduce raw and cold foods.

> Avoid foods you don't digest well.
> Add in small amounts of fermented foods or try taking a probiotic supplement.
> Use longer cooking times with moderate heat. Try steaming, simmering, and poaching, and eat more soups and stews.
> Aim for simple food preparation and combinations and moderation in all flavors.
> Add naturally sweet foods, such as whole grains, easy-to-digest legumes like split yellow mung beans, stewed fruit, dates, and vegetables like snap peas, parsnips, and squash.
> Seek out foods that are yellow or orange like millet, yams, carrots, corn, pumpkins, and sweet potatoes.
> Avoid excessively hot, heavy, and oily foods; they can aggravate accumulated heat from summer. Reduce foods that are difficult to digest, cause inflammation, or are Damp-forming, like dairy and sugar.
> If you're in late summer and moving closer to autumn, add more sour foods like grapes, apples, rose hips, and pomegranates.
> Herbal medicines should focus on supporting your digestive capacity and preparing the body for the cooler months. Use herbs like ginger root (*sheng jiang*), coix seed (*yi yi ren*), and Chinese licorice root (*gan cao*) to strengthen digestion and clear Dampness. To support overall energy and nourish your Heart and digestive capacity, try the herbal formula Restore the Spleen Decoction (*Gui Pi Tang*). You'll want to avoid this formula if there are Heat signs in your body. Lastly, the Ayurvedic remedy commonly called CCF (cumin, coriander, fennel) is a wonderful option; use it after big meals to improve digestion and absorption or periodically for a few days to boost your system. To make it, bring three cups of water to a boil; add 1 tablespoon each of cumin, coriander, and fennel seeds. Turn the heat down, cover, and simmer for 10 minutes. Remove from heat and allow to steep 10 minutes longer. Strain and drink throughout the day.

As you can see, Earth is our rooted center and represents a flourishing time. Along with seasonal changes, we can also get to know how this element supports our bodies and minds. Now we'll look at the subtle body organs and meridians, then in the following two chapters we'll investigate how our Earth element comes alive with emotion and spirit.

ORGANS OF THE EARTH ELEMENT

In the Chinese medical map of the body, the nourishing late summer and Earth element relate to the energetic organs of the Spleen and Stomach. We need a way to process and assimilate all the golden Earth element abundance we've been exploring—physically, mentally, emotionally, energetically, and spiritually—and these organs do just that. Please note that on a physical level, some of the functions Chinese medicine attributes to the energetic Spleen are more closely related to the physical organ of the pancreas, so I will touch on both here (in Western medicine, the pancreas is not directly related to the spleen).

Physically, the spleen and pancreas play crucial roles in maintaining the body's overall health, with the spleen primarily involved in the immune system and blood filtration and the pancreas contributing to digestion and blood sugar regulation. Your spleen is about the size of a fist and lies on the upper left side of your abdomen, beneath your rib cage. It filters blood, removes damaged blood cells, and stores platelets. It also plays a vital role in your immune system—it traps bacteria and houses white blood cells to fight infection. Your pancreas is a flat, elongated gland that rests a little to the right of center in your upper abdomen behind your stomach. It produces and secretes digestive enzymes into the small intestine to aid in the digestion of carbohydrates, fats, and proteins, and it releases hormones into the bloodstream to regulate blood sugar levels. The stomach, the Earth element's paired Yang organ, sits near the middle of your abdomen, just to the left. It receives food and expands and shrinks in size depending on the amount of food it holds. The stomach secretes hydrochloric acid and enzymes, and with the help of peristaltic movements, it mixes food and contributes to the process of digestion and assimilation before moving food along for further processing in the small intestine.

In Chinese medicine, these organs hold immense importance for their contribution to digestion. I always tell my patients and students that, like the Earth element in the center of the Five Element model, digestion is truly at the center of health. When our Earth element is balanced, we literally feel earthy—grounded, sated, rich, and alive. On the other hand, every cell in the body-mind will suffer if we can't break down and assimilate the nutrients and vital life force (or Qi) held within food. Without healthy Earth element organs, we feel dull and weak. And remember, digestion refers to food and the body, but also the processing of thoughts and experiences in the mind, which we'll explore in Chapter 12.

Energetically, your Spleen and Stomach transport food through the digestive tract and transform it into usable energy. These organs are responsible for the entire process from the moment you desire food, based on your appetite, to the release of enzymes and the eventual mechanical breakdown of food particles. They're even in control of your knowing which types of foods will truly nourish you. The Stomach receives food, draws some fluids out, starts the breakdown process, and then sends it downward. In Chinese medicine, we say it's the official in charge of "rotting and ripening." If this function isn't working, we may experience stagnation, rebellious Stomach Qi (when Stomach Qi moves in the wrong direction), or Stomach Fire or Cold, any of which could lead to ulcers, heartburn, nausea, stomach fullness or pain, vomiting, burping, or hiccupping.

The Yin organ of the pair, the Spleen, is the energetic organ that is least like its Western counterpart. Remember, we primarily define Chinese medicine organs in relation to their energetic functions rather than their anatomical location, which is especially true of the energetic Spleen. In Chinese medicine, the Spleen assists the Stomach in transforming and transporting nutritive food essences to the body, much like the body sending glucose to cells for energy. For example, when cells have poor insulin uptake, as in the case of insulin resistance, we may experience fatigue and cravings for sweet foods, which are classic indicators of Spleen Qi depletion. The energetic Spleen also sends food Qi to the energetic Lungs and the Heart to assist in the formation of Blood, eventually nourishing all our tissues. Blood, created through the digestive process, is the primary vehicle for Qi to circulate throughout the body. Without Blood and Qi, the body cannot build itself or heal. When our Spleen Qi is healthy, we have strong muscles and limbs, and our Blood is nutrient-dense. If a patient of mine has feeble muscles, is exhausted, or is pale, I make a note to assess their Earth element and digestive capacity.

In TCM, the Spleen is responsible for "raising Qi" and controlling Blood overall, so if you experience Qi moving downward in the body when it shouldn't (say as a prolapse anywhere in the body), have excessive bleeding, or bruise easily, this is a sign your Spleen Qi may be weak. The Earth element is also related to your mouth, lips, and sense of taste. Bad breath, mouth sores, bleeding gums, and pale or cracked lips often indicate Earth element imbalance. The mouth is where we receive food, and many link it unconsciously to our first experiences of nourishment and comfort through breastfeeding. Later in life this sense organ, if it's healthy, can help us decipher whether something will nourish and feed us or be harmful, hard to digest, or even poisonous. When our Earth element is healthy, we have a balanced relationship with food and the comfort it provides; our cravings and choices are right for us, we can taste all flavors, and we produce saliva appropriately. My patients with eating disorders usually need to work on Earth element issues to heal their relationship with food. However, the most common signs of low Spleen Qi are fatigue and digestive symptoms—especially a weak appetite, food sensitivities, bloating, and loose stools (explored in the next chapter).

EARTH ELEMENT MERIDIANS

Along with the Earth element organs, we can also tap into the power of the energetic meridians of the Spleen and Stomach. The Sinew channels for the Spleen begin on the medial edges of your big toes and run up the inner legs and thighs to the groin, abdomen, and navel with branches to your ribs, chest, and spine. The primary meridians also travel to the upper chest, where they descend and terminate on the sides of the torso beneath your armpits. The Stomach Sinew meridians start on the tops of your feet at the middle three toes and travel up the fronts of your legs to your hip joints, pelvic region, lower ribs, and spine. From there, they ascend your abdomen, chest, neck, and face with branches near your ears and eyes. The primary meridians also run near the hairline. Postures and movements that target these areas help harmonize the flow of Qi through these subtle body channels.

To support these channels and subtler meridians associated with the energetic Spleen and Stomach—and the Earth element in general—we can choose specific movements and yoga postures that target the tissues at the fronts of the legs, the abdomen, and the inner thighs. In postural dynamics, a common imbalance occurs when the front body sags down or draws in, and the back body seems to lift up. This posture can contribute to sluggish digestion and a feeling of heaviness and lethargy common with Earth element imbalance. Movements that lengthen the myofascial bands at the front body that contribute to that pattern, such as backbends, are particularly helpful in reestablishing balance.

Sensing the Earth Element Channels and Organs in Saddle or Supta Virasana (Reclining Hero Pose)

Begin by sitting on your heels with your knees apart; place a bolster behind you. Lean back on your hands, then lie back so your spine is supported on the bolster. If you have the range of motion, you can remove the bolster and lie on the floor. If these options are not accessible for your knees or hips, try placing your feet beside your outer hips (Virasana) and using more height, such as a soft block or two or a couple of stacked blankets, under your sitting bones. Placing a blanket behind your knees is also a nice option. From there, you can stay upright or recline back onto your hands or a bolster or two. If none of these variations work, you can do this practice lying on your back directly on the floor.

Once you are adequately set up, gently draw your sacrum away from your lumbar vertebrae and relax.

Soften your breath and begin to visualize your Earth element meridians. Allow your mind to trace your Spleen meridians from your big toes up your inner legs to your abdomen, then your Stomach channels from the tops of your feet to the fronts of your legs and up your torso. As you trace these pathways, notice any sensations from the posture, like tugging or pressure on the tissues. Stay patiently with the sensations for a couple of minutes.

Next, bring your awareness to your digestive organs. These organs, which lie just below your respiratory diaphragm, can either work together or become overly burdened. If it helps, you can place your hands on this area. Feel any internal sensations. As you inhale, you may feel your diaphragm gently pressing these organs down, and as you exhale, you may feel this whole area reorganizing as the diaphragm moves up.

Yellow is the color we associate with these organs of nourishment and Earth Qi. As you breathe, imagine a bright yellow color imbuing your Spleen, Stomach, and Pancreas with energy. Stay visualizing this color for 5 to 10 breaths. To exit the pose, relax any concentration and use your hands to push yourself up. Take your time extending your legs out in front of you. Contract your quadriceps by lifting your knees a few times before moving on.

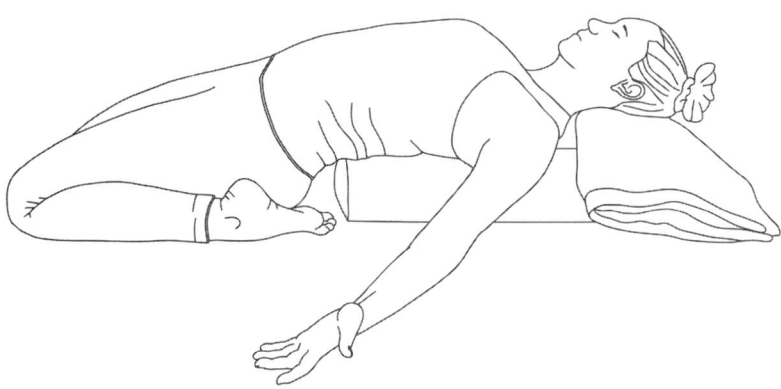

ELEVEN

NOURISH CENTER

Sit like a mountain. Sit with a sense of strength and dignity. Be steadfast, be majestic, be natural, and at ease in awareness. No matter how many winds are blowing, no matter how many clouds are swirling, no matter how many lions are prowling, be intimate with everything and sit like a mountain.[32]
—SHARON SALZBERG

The Earth element manifests its full, luxurious, and pleasant energy in nature, in the seasons, and in our bodies through our organs, tissues, and energetic channels. Earth nourishes us with abundant bounty, but it can get weighed down with too much processing if we're not careful. Let's look at some common ways we get out of balance and practices to help.

EARTH ELEMENT CONGESTION

When people begin to pay more attention to their physical health, one of the first places they often discover imbalance is in the digestive system. Gut health is the nucleus of overall health; attending to and healing Earth element imbalances in the gastrointestinal region, or GI tract, is vital for whole body-mind health. Conditions involving the gut can be complex, and we need to tailor solutions to the individual; nonetheless, there are some basic principles and practices you can follow that will help.

In my clinical practice and teaching, I regularly see patients and students with weak digestion (often indicating Spleen Qi deficiency), leading to the formation of Dampness. Internal Dampness is a Yin energy that is sticky, heavy, wet, and sometimes cold. It forms when the Earth element and digestion can't transform what was meant to nourish us. Dampness is similar in some ways to the Ayurvedic concept of *ama*, a buildup of toxic residue often caused by poor digestive and metabolic breakdown. The symptoms of internal Dampness vary because it can affect many locations and functions. Still, general symptoms indicate stagnation and mucus buildup in the organs, particularly in the digestive system. In my practice, patients in this category most often have trouble digesting a wide range of foods and experience bloating, fatigue, brain fog, and weight gain; others have been diagnosed with food sensitivities, dysbiosis, irritable bowel syndrome, and even cysts or tumors (which are usually a combination of Blood stasis and Phlegm—an advanced stage of Dampness).

It helps to think of your digestion and Earth element as a soup pot over a campfire—you want to keep the fire just right to cook the soup evenly. If the logs are too damp, the flames go out. Feed the flame too often or with the wrong kind of logs, and the soup doesn't cook correctly. In Ayurveda, we say this fire of digestion relies on agni. Related to the English word "ignite," agni is the force of intelligence within each cell; it is the spark that governs absorption, assimilation, and transportation. Ultimately, the goal is to have a digestive system that burns clean, with no leftover residue, to create strong, resilient tissues.

Physically, the GI tract is a long tube that runs from the mouth to the anus and includes the esophagus, stomach, and small and large intestines. It receives and breaks down food and liquids through the release of enzymes and hormones, as well as muscle movement. It releases nutrients and energy into the body and eliminates waste. The GI tract is so special that it is sometimes called the second, enteric, or gut brain because of its beautiful and intricate functions. Did you know that millions of neurons inside your gut sense and receive elaborate impulses and are influenced by your nervous system, emotions, and memory? Or that about 80 percent of your immune system lives in the gut? It is also home to an ecosystem unique to you. It contains trillions of bacteria, fungi, viruses, and yeast, which we call your gut flora or microbiota. Many of these microbes coevolved with humans over millennia and live harmoniously or symbiotically with you. Studying these microbes is still an emerging science, but it's a growing field of research with some exciting possibilities.

Your microbiome (including all microorganisms living in and on your body) begins at birth. Inside the womb, a fetus is wholly protected and isolated from these microbes, but during a routine vaginal birth, colonization begins. A newborn is covered in Mom's flora as the baby moves through the birth canal and receives bacteria from the environment and from skin-to-skin contact during cuddling and kissing. C-section babies still pick up bacteria over time, but their GI tract and immune system generally take longer to colonize. Eventually, breastfeeding also contributes to a baby's microbial biodiversity. These initial bacteria are the first to colonize our digestive system. They reproduce quickly and constantly change through exposure to new microorganisms. They also shape the foundations of our immune system. In Chinese medicine, this forms part of our postnatal Qi, the energy we receive from our food and environment that determines a big part of our overall strength and digestive capacity.

The neurons and bacteria in your gut are integral to you and profoundly influence your mental and physical health. If you've ever had the stomach flu, you've experienced how unfriendly bacteria somehow made their way into your food or water and wreaked havoc. But most bacteria that live inside us are harmless; in fact, we need them. Beneficial microbes in your body help you break down difficult-to-digest foods, supply you with energy, train your immune system, make vitamins, and break down medications and toxins. Some bacteria are responsible for blood groups; some make things like gases, fats, and acids. The more diversity in this ecosystem of microbes, the better. About 80 percent of the body's serotonin and up to 50 percent of its dopamine are in the gut.[33] Serotonin helps with digestion, learning, sleep, mood, feelings of self-worth, sexual desire, and bone health. Dopamine is involved in reward and motivation. Studies even link gut bacteria imbalances to obesity, nervous disorders, anxiety, depression, malnutrition, and chronic digestive issues, among many other concerns.

What's fantastic is that modern science is catching up to what holistic systems have known all along: digestion is at the core of many health concerns. In fact, holistic systems tell us that caring for digestion is one of the easiest ways to maintain health and longevity. A healthy microbiome and gut flora mean excellent digestion, energy, and a stable Earth element. When your microbes work optimally, your body can break down and assimilate food and nutrients and eliminate toxins and waste efficiently. Plus, your immune system will be ready when you face challenges. Poor nutrition, soil depletion, inflammation, stress, and frequent use of antibiotics can negatively impact these helpful bacteria and, therefore, Earth element vitality.

To have a healthy Earth element and digestion, we need good elimination, and we need to consume the right kinds of foods in the right amounts, at the correct times, and in the right way for our condition, constitution, age, and season. Digestive disorders and Dampness are usually tricky to treat because Dampness doesn't usually change quickly. Many students and patients who come to me to heal and strengthen their digestion have been struggling with concerns for years and have cut out many foods in an attempt to remedy weak digestive capacity. While cutting out trigger foods can be helpful in the short term—and I often employ different elimination diets with patients—it's not the whole picture, nor is it usually a long-term solution.

I typically use a three-step approach with my patients. First, we determine the foods and lifestyle choices contributing to the imbalance and try to cut out what is throwing the body out of balance—at least for a time. Which foods, activities, and substances nourish and which ones harm depends on your unique sensitivities, needs, and constitutional makeup.

Next, we work on healing any damage done and restoring the gut to its natural balance. We do this with specific healing foods, herbal medicines, practices, and sometimes supplements like probiotics.

Well-cooked foods are helpful if digestion is weak, and if your system can handle digesting them, fermented foods and fiber-rich prebiotic foods such as lentils, beans, dandelion greens, or artichokes also support balance. There are many medicinal foods and herbal medicines beyond the scope of this book that I use in my practice. Those healing remedies are primary keys in helping many of my patients heal gut disorders. This stage takes time as we need to give the mucous lining of the gut and the microbiome plenty of opportunity to repair. Finally, when the gut is in a healthier state, we may be able to reintroduce some of the foods that were cut out, albeit in smaller amounts or with more mindful awareness of their effects on the body-mind.

Change can be difficult, especially when it comes to food. When modern society inundates us with unhealthy processed and packaged food, it can sometimes feel impossible to know how to choose what's best, but here's the thing: You don't need to become excessively picky about food to regain health. Nutrition and detailed food choices are a huge topic, but despite how confusing the world of nutrition can be, holistic systems highlight a way of eating that is actually quite simple. Initially, I guide patients and students in choosing fresh, seasonal, whole, natural, and preferably organic foods to support good gut health. Humans have always eaten this way, across all cultures, and I've found it is the most sustainable choice for most people in the long term. I love Michael Pollan's saying, "Eat food. Not too much. Mostly plants." A diet like that builds robust Qi and Blood, evens out blood sugar, supports immunity and hormones, reduces inflammation, and so much more.

High-quality whole foods like vegetables, whole grains, legumes, beans, nuts, seeds, healthy oils, fruit, seaweed, natural sweeteners, and small amounts of probiotic foods will give your body plenty of life-giving Qi, vitamins, and minerals for peak function and good digestion. This diet also automatically eliminates foods that are specifically bad for your gut. Of course, if you have specific health concerns, preferences, or limitations, I suggest tweaking your foundational diet with your health care provider using remedies, techniques, and practices for specific imbalances.

Habits for Healthy Digestion

Healing and strengthening your Earth element and improving digestion are about much more than just the food you eat. If you want to build your digestive strength and clear any Damp residue that has built up, here are a few habits to implement right away:

> › Create regular and consistent routines around cooking, mealtimes, and meal preparation.
> › Relax when eating as much as possible. Sit down to eat in a peaceful environment with limited distractions. Chew well.
> › Monitor your hunger. Your appetite is a natural response you can tune in to to discover what your body needs. Pay attention to when you feel hungry and when you feel full. Don't ignore your hunger and don't overeat.
> › Eat during daylight and enjoy your biggest meal midday.
> › Allow time and space between meals. Try to avoid a lot of snacking. This can take some time to adjust to, so go slow and add longer-lasting fats and proteins to your meals to sustain energy.
> › Drink warm water between meals.
> › Enjoy your food! Pleasure toward eating will help your digestive capacity. Linger and savor your meal's flavors and aromas.

TASTING NOURISHMENT

The sensory organ most closely linked to the Earth element is the mouth, with its connection to eating and nourishment. Use the preceding and following recommendations to find balance.

How to Break Up with Sugar

The flavor linked to the Earth element is sweet. Now before you start in on that next piece of pie to heal your Earth element, hold on. I'm talking about foods that are *naturally* sweet and taste more moderate, such as carrots, sweet potatoes, corn, and even whole grains. Sweet foods are at the center of our diet because they're the foods our bodies need most often. They're nourishing and building—complex carbohydrates; lots of veggies; even legumes, some meats, and dairy are a little energetically sweet.

I probably don't have to tell you that too much refined or processed sugar in your diet is a different story. Too much sugar depletes your body over time. Along with all the health impacts you already know about, excess processed sugar is the worst thing for your Earth element. To add insult to injury, if your Earth is out of balance, it's often the one thing you crave the most. Quitting processed sugar can be tough, but I help patients and students do it all the time. It is possible! No need to quit sweet treats completely, but I do recommend cutting way back on refined sugar and sticking to alternatives instead. To help you make this shift, here are a few tips I give my students and patients:

> Clear it out. Eliminate processed sugar from your home completely. Clean out your cupboards, fridge, and vehicle. If it's not there, it won't tempt you.
> Make sure your blood sugar stays stable throughout the day. Eat high-quality fat or protein at every meal, and never get to the point where you're "hangry." Always keep a few nutrient-dense snacks around for those times when you need a pick-me-up right away.
> Drink enough water. Often cravings are actually masking dehydration.
> Cook at home. It's difficult to control the amount of hidden sugar you're getting at restaurants and cafés.
> Eat other foods that have a sweet flavor when you really need a fix. These foods may not seem sweet at first, but gradually, you'll acquire a more refined taste. Try fruit, yams, carrots, licorice tea, cinnamon, beets, and squash to get started. A small amount of dark chocolate (70 percent or higher) will also curb your craving—just don't overdo it!

> Replace old habits with new ones. If you're used to always having a sweet treat after dinner, create a new habit of doing 10 minutes of stretching, reading, or knitting instead. If you usually have a sugary pick-me-up midday, replace the habit with a walk around the block.

Healing Congee

This simple, thin porridge makes a perfect healing remedy for gut health. In TCM we say it helps supplement Speen Qi and Blood because it is so nourishing and easy to digest. Use it when weak from illness, the day after a big meal, or anytime your digestion needs a break. Traditionally this dish is made with rice, although you can also use a variety of other grains. Adding vegetables, legumes, herbal medicines, or other spices can also provide variety and specific healing properties.

½ cup brown rice, rinsed well
4–6 cups water
pinch of salt and ginger powder

Bring water to a boil; add the rice, ginger, and salt. You can also add ground cinnamon and dried fruit for a sweet breakfast congee, or make a savory version with spices like fennel, black pepper, turmeric, or ground cumin. Turn the heat down, cover, and simmer for 1–4 hours. A crockpot also works well. The grains will split and the dish will become more watery the longer the cook time. The longer congee cooks, the more powerful and easier to digest it becomes. Remove from heat and serve.

PRACTICES FOR BALANCE

Movements and practices that support digestion; strengthen the body's big muscles; or build stability in the feet, knees, and legs create grounding and connection to the Earth element, as do movements that introduce mobility in the hip joints and sacrum. Standing yoga postures with a focus on the out-breath, which we explore here, are particularly well suited to support this element. You can also use balance postures and movements that engage your abdominal muscles to build a little heat to stoke your digestive fire and twists to release stagnation. In yoga, we call this activating *samana vayu*, which is an energetic movement connected to the Fire element. If you experience irregularity or spasmodic pain tied to digestion, opt for restorative forward bends and avoid stimulating postures that put excess pressure on the abdomen.

Belly Massage

Use this practice when you feel your digestion is congested, or try it anytime to tune in to your digestive fire.

Begin by finding a comfortable position, either lying down or seated. Place your hands on your abdomen just below your ribs with your fingers pointing in. Sweep your hands clockwise around your abdomen while gently pressing down. You can also gently shake your hands as you press downward and move them in a circular fashion around your navel. Breathe slowly in a relaxed way. Continue moving in a circular motion two to three more times. Afterward, rest your palms on your lower abdomen for 2 to 5 minutes, sensing into the center of your belly.

Grounding Stance with Gushing Spring

Many martial arts, such as Tai Ji and Qi Gong, use a standing meditation stance to help practitioners develop strength in their legs and a sense of firm balance. In some ways, this stance is similar to the yoga postures of Tadasana (Mountain Pose) or Samasthiti (Equal Standing Pose). There are many ways to practice a grounding stance, depending on the tradition you are following, but the basic premise remains the same: the position should help you find your rooted center in a comfortable and natural way.

In this practice, we'll explore a stance I first learned during a time I spent studying Chinese medicine nutrition with Paul Pitchford, in the rolling hills of beautiful Northern California many years ago. Aside from his remarkable teaching and guidance regarding food, I also had the pleasure of witnessing his true passion for Tai Ji. We would regularly move through a series of postures to open our energetic channels and prepare us for the day's studies, always beginning with some form of a grounding stance to root and connect our energies to the power of the earth beneath us. Use this practice to strengthen your Earth element, ground your mind, and find more balance.

To start this practice, ideally find a place to stand outside barefoot; if that's not possible, practicing indoors is fine. Begin by standing with your feet slightly wider than hip-width apart and softly bend your knees. Once you've found this basic setup, try varying your stance to make it a little wider or narrower until you find a comfortable and natural position. Distribute your weight equally between your feet and press firmly (but not forcefully) down into the earth. To create a stronger sense of grounding, bend your knees more deeply so your body and center of gravity are lower. Allow your spine to be upright, and soften your gaze. Remember, the aim here is a feeling of natural steadiness. Keep experimenting with the exact stance until you feel comfortable.

Once you have found an appropriate stance, move your awareness into your lower body. Visualize your Qi dropping into your legs and feet. If your legs are too tense to feel energy circulating, create more ease by straightening your knees a little. Feel and sense the supportive and receptive ground beneath you. Where do you feel contact with the earth? As you settle in, imagine your legs and feet slowly growing a strong taproot and eventually smaller secondary roots off the sides. Feel how this root system supports you in becoming more stable and balanced.

At the base of your foot (between the second and third toes, approximately one-third the distance between the base of the second toe and the heel) is an energetic point called Gushing Spring (*Yong Quan*) in TCM or Foot Middle (*Pada Madhya*) in Ayurvedic marma. This point is on the Kidney meridian, but because it is the lowest point on the body, it is a powerful doorway into Earth energy. Visualize this point and gently concentrate on it to descend and ground your energy.

As your body roots downward and becomes more centered, encourage your mind to do the same. Stay for 2 to 5 minutes, steadying your posture and your mind.

Supported Virabhadrasana II (Warrior II Pose) with Pada Bandha (Foot Lock)

Using a chair for this posture helps to reduce muscular effort so you can experience a greater sense of grounding and opening of your feet, legs, and pelvis. It's ideal for those looking to build strength, improve hip flexibility, or relieve pressure in the knees or lower back.

Choose a sturdy chair without arms and place it on a stable surface. Begin by straddling the back of the chair with one foot on either side. Place your left foot on the floor with your knee bent at a 90-degree angle and your foot pointing away from the chair. Straighten your right leg in the opposite direction, turning your foot at an angle toward the chair. You should now be in the basic form for Virabhadrasana II, with your torso and hips facing the back of the chair and your legs on either side. Root your buttocks decisively into the chair and your feet firmly into the floor. If your feet don't reach the floor, place support like a hardcover book or yoga block under each one until they have full contact. Place support under your pelvis if the chair is too low or your legs are longer. Maintain even weight distribution across both sitting bones for stability.

Stretch your right leg by pressing through your outer heel and lifting your knee to engage your quadriceps. Press down through your left foot as you roll your front knee outward. Press your hands on the back of the chair, and continue to lift your abdomen and turn it toward the back of the chair. From this position, you can focus on an energetic engagement we call Pada Bandha in yoga. Pada Bandha involves lifting from the centers of your feet while remaining grounded, encouraging energy to move up the legs. Press the four corners of each foot down and try to lift your arches. Keep your legs active as you remain in the pose, feeling a sense of Earth energy for a few minutes. Switch legs and repeat on the opposite side.

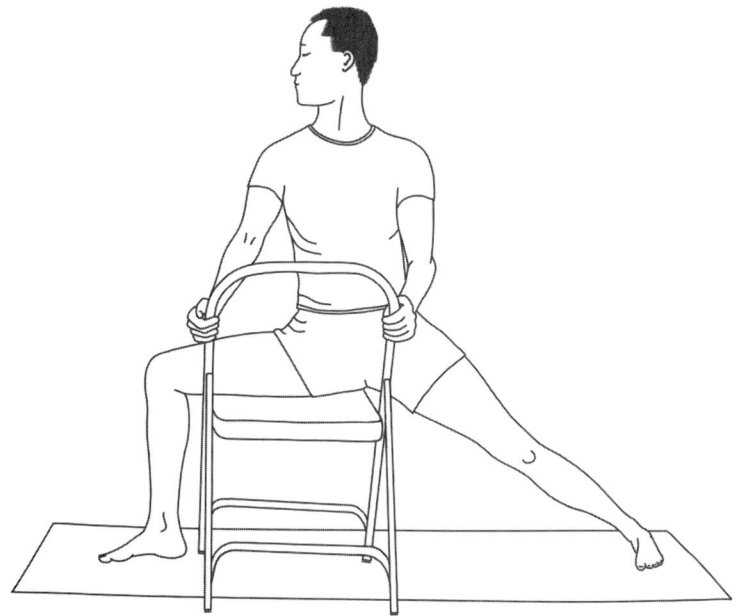

Utkatasana (Fierce Pose or Chair Pose) with Block

———

Utkatasana encourages a strong focus on leg engagement, especially in the large, blood-filled muscles of the quadriceps where the Spleen and Stomach meridians run. Adding the block helps gather energy and attention at the body's midline, enhancing a sense of centering and focus.

Begin in a standing position. Place a yoga block between your upper thighs, just above the knees. Squeeze the block so it fits snugly between your legs. Then bend your knees, lowering your hips as if sitting back in a chair. Continue to squeeze the block so you can feel engagement in your inner thighs and a steady lower body. Allow your torso to lean slightly forward, inviting a gentle arch in your lower back. Relax your toes. Press the four corners of each foot into the floor and lift your arches. Hold the pose for a few breaths focusing on the exhale. Keep your thighs active and your inner leg muscles engaged with the block. To release, exhale, push into your feet, and straighten your legs.

Belly Breathing with the Field of Elixir

Belly Breathing is a great daily practice to connect with a sense of ease and stability in your "home base"—the Earth element at your center. This practice also releases stagnation in your respiratory diaphragm and digestive organs. During a healthy, full breath, the dome-shaped muscle of the respiratory diaphragm alternately contracts and relaxes, pushing on and releasing the digestive organs beneath it. The area we'll be focusing on is a critical energetic center in Daoism and yoga. In Chinese medicine, the area between the navel and pelvic floor is called the Field of Elixir (lower *Dan Tian*). Settling awareness downward into this field helps us remain grounded and centered in our bodies and minds. Martial artists use concentration on this area to establish a strong foundation when an opponent is trying to topple them. In yoga, this area as a whole relates to the lower energetic centers connected to our physicality, security, and personal power. Without a connection to this energetic center, we lose our anchor to the Earth element and our sense of personal psychological and spiritual ground.

To begin this practice, lie on your back with your knees bent and your feet on the floor, allowing your knees to fall toward one another. Bring your hands to your lower abdomen, just below your navel. Notice any gripping or tightening. It's common to discover bracing and stagnation in and around the belly, especially if you have a history of trauma or you've internalized the message to suck in your abdomen for appearances. Remember, whether you feel a sense of vitality or numbness and gripping when you try this practice, your Earth energy life force is there supporting you. Simply bringing awareness to this area is an essential first step in healing any divide you experience.

Breathe slowly and softly through your nostrils. Notice if your abdomen balloons outward as you inhale and recedes inward as you exhale. Next, encourage your breath to gently deepen and lengthen to about a 5- or 6-second in-breath and out-breath. As you breathe, observe the expansion and contraction of your ribs, including your upper, side, and lower ribs. Then imagine your breath moving down into your belly. As you breathe in, notice your abdomen rising, and as you breathe out, watch it fall. Patiently return to observing your breath in your belly if your mind wanders. This practice is more about releasing than doing anything. Allow yourself to relax and continue to gently attend to your breath. Practice this technique regularly, especially if you are healing Earth element imbalances.

If you want to expand on this practice, visualize a ball of energy inside your abdomen as you breathe. On the inhalation, you might imagine the ball growing slightly larger. As you exhale, visualize the ball returning to its original size. Practice this method for 5 to 10 minutes, then release all effort and return to a natural breath without visualization.

Nadi Shodhana Pranayama (Channel Purifying Breath)

This breath practice is commonly used in yoga to cleanse and balance the subtle energetic channels. In modern terms, there is some evidence to show that it helps balance the nervous system and the activity of the brain's two hemispheres. Since the Earth element is all about balance, this practice is perfect for harmonizing Earth element Qi.

To practice, find a comfortable seat. Soften your eyes. This practice is traditionally done using a hand gesture called Mrigi Mudra (Deer Seal), but here we will use a simplified version of the hands to focus on the breathing technique. Feel free to use the original mudra if you are familiar with it. For the simplified version, take your dominant hand and curl your pinkie finger into the palm. Place your middle and index fingers (I call these our "peace fingers") between your eyebrows and slightly bend your ring finger. Rest your opposite hand on your leg. Relax your neck and shoulders. As you settle into your seat, exhale fully through both nostrils. Then place the tip of your thumb in the small hollow on the side of your nostril to block air passage. Do not forcefully press the nostril closed; instead, envision your fingertips as sensitive receptors, using the correct pressure to close the airway without pushing the nose out of shape.

Let's use the right hand as an example of one round: Close the right nostril with your thumb and inhale through your left nostril. Next, unblock your right nostril and block your left nostril with your ring finger. Exhale through your right nostril. Continue blocking the left side and inhale through the right nostril. To conclude, block your right nostril and exhale through the left. Try starting this practice with four to five rounds at once and eventually increase the number to nine rounds daily.

In this chapter, we explored the organs of the Earth element, some of the physical ailments that arise from Earth element imbalances, and some habits and practices to harmonize Earth. In the next chapter, we'll move on to its subtle aspects, including emotional and spiritual imbalance and associated practices.

TWELVE

GROUNDED INTENTION

The highest function of earth is to nourish all creatures
without partiality which is the acme of good faith.
—BAI HU TONG

Earth is our grounded center. Its power is in assimilating and transforming torrential rain, the heat of the sun, and the decay of fallen
grasses and great trees into something nourishing and life-giving. In our
bodies, it digests the food we eat, and in our minds, it helps us process
the thoughts we have. The Earth element is responsible for integrating the stuff of our lives in a way that will be nourishing for us. In fact,
everything we take in daily, as well as everything we have experienced in
our lives, requires a breakdown and absorption. When we have a healthy
Earth element, we're able to receive and process what has happened to
us and turn it into life lessons. Our traumas and joys get "digested" and
transformed into "nutrition" that feeds our understanding of ourselves
and our place in the world. That takes place on a physical level, as is the
case when we digest food, and on a psychological or emotional level,
as is the case when we take in everything we experience, read, watch,
or hear. Without a healthy Earth element, we're not able to break down
what we consume into usable parts. We not only have trouble digesting
food, but we also lose our center and have difficulty receiving nourishment from life.

From the perspective of Chinese medicine, mental digestion happens
when we concentrate, think, create ideas, and mull things over. When

your Earth element is out of balance, it will cause excessive rumination and worry—the negative emotions and mental states most closely associated with the Earth element. In TCM, we say these states cause Qi to knot because they generally move around and around with no resulting action or forward direction. Over time, Qi gets all twisted up with this circular movement. Remember, thought itself is not the problem; it only becomes pathological when we *overthink* things. The connection between thoughts and digestion even plays out in our language. Perhaps there's something that's "eating you," that you're "chewing on," something you can't quite "stomach," or maybe you're "worried sick." We all know when faced with an experience we can't quite digest, thinking about it over and over doesn't generally help.

When we worry, are anxious, or ruminate, we lose connection to our body and the sense of ground beneath us and become trapped in an endless cycle of the mind. From the perspective of Chinese medicine, it takes energy to overthink, so Qi is directed away from our digestive system and all-knowing Heart. I find it fascinating how often my patients who have concerns about physical digestive issues also experience overthinking or anxiety—especially considering all we explored in the previous chapter regarding the link between the gut microbiome and mental health. This imbalance can also manifest if you have too many mental tasks on your plate. I remember when I was studying in school, my classmates and I often gave each other acupuncture for Earth element depletion, which was almost invariably caused by too much studying. In TCM, this connection between mind and body can go either way; a long-standing physical imbalance can lead to emotional changes, or repressed or deeply held emotions can lead to physical imbalance. In any case, if you worry a lot, get caught in overthinking, or are involved in tasks that take excessive mental activity, you most certainly want to strengthen your overall digestive capacity by focusing on the Earth element.

We largely base our thinking on what we consume, so the first step in healing this aspect of Earth element imbalance is to be discerning about what you take in in the first place. Second, you'll need to make sure you're externally and internally nourished and grounded enough to be able to process and assimilate whatever comes your way. This involves eating foods that sustain you, which we covered in the last chapter, and balancing your needs with the needs of others, which we'll explore later in this chapter. Third, to heal the Earth element specifically—and access its spiritual gifts—you can work with your thoughts directly to transform them into heart-centered intention, integrity, habit, and service. This requires you to stay centered and steady like a humble farmer, one who shows up daily to receive from and give to the earth with patience and dedication.

THE SPIRIT OF EARTH

On a psychospiritual level, Yi, which translates as "intent" or "thought," is the state of consciousness or aspect of awareness that represents the Earth element. Specifically, Yi is at the very root of our thoughts and forms the basis of our thinking. The TCM scholar Elisabeth Rochat calls this quality our "inner disposition." I love this interpretation because it captures both how we view the world and how we behave. The Chinese character for Yi contains two parts. One portrays a mouth with a sound coming out, such as a spoken word or music; the other is the character for the Heart.[34] When aligned, Yi expresses the Heart's sound or intention. The *Nei Jing* states, "When the heart reflects on something, that is called Yi (intention)."[35] In yoga, we call this *sankalpa*, a higher heartfelt vow. You may remember from our exploration of the Fire element that the concepts of Heart and mind are very similar. So when I say that the Yi is expressing your Heart song, you could say it's expressing your mind's song too.

We explored earlier how the role of the Earth element is to metabolize what we consume both physically and mentally. From a psychological perspective, everything you take in eventually gets digested, affects your thoughts, and influences your eventual intentions. Yi represents your intentions that arise from your thoughts and beliefs, which are formed based on everything you digest. In Confucian philosophy, Yi is also one of four crucial virtues that occur naturally when a person lives in harmony with the earth, others, and their Dao. When your intentions are healthy, you live and act with integrity based on an awareness of reciprocity.

Classical texts invite us to consciously cultivate Yi by first getting to the root of negative mind states and then working to increase skillful ones. For example, if you continually surround yourself with people who speak with violence, jealousy, or hatred, your mind and thoughts could easily become tainted by those qualities. If, instead, you seek out people who influence you with messages of inspiration or hope, you will be more inclined toward altruism, compassion, and joy. The Buddha's well-known teaching from the *Dhammapada* outlines the connection between our deeper intentions and our actions succinctly:

> Phenomena are preceded by the heart, ruled by the heart, made of the heart. If you speak or act with a corrupted heart, then suffering follows you—as the wheel of the cart, the track of the ox that pulls it . . . If you speak or act with a calm, bright heart, then happiness follows you, like a shadow that never leaves.[36]

In particular, the Chinese classics suggest that we study books written by wise teachers and spend time in nature contemplating the movement of seasons and other natural phenomena to help nourish and purify the Heart-Mind and clarify our understanding of reality.

We often speak and act without thinking, out of habit or conditioning, and without any clear intention. However, taking in things that nourish us feeds a clear view, and therefore our Yi will help us act with integrity and steadily move us toward what is truly good for us. In Buddhism, these characteristics are essential pillars on the eightfold path: right view, thought, and action. Practicing them gives you more clarity of mind, and you're less likely to chase after empty pleasures. Your worries can subside, and you may experience heightened feelings of generosity, satiety, and abundance—all qualities of good Earth element Qi. When this happens, you can still have goals, but those goals are informed by your deeper values. We'll explore those concepts more in the practice section of this chapter.

Rarely will doing something once make a significant impact on our lives. Instead, when our Yi is healthy, we harness its power through repetitive action aligned with our intentions. Earth stays consistent in the moment but changes over time. For example, you're not likely to see a big difference if you eat a healthy meal once or work on a new project for one day. You must continue to do the thing until it becomes a regular habit; only then will you truly experience the impact of having a healthy Yi. When rooted in steady faithfulness, Yi helps you be like a caring, dependable, and loyal gardener—devoted to your fertile ground, consistent with your habits, and aligned with your Heart's calling. In fact, we need our good intentions to sustain any regular practice, such as yoga or meditation. When our motives, thoughts, and actions lack healthy Earth qualities, we live ungrounded and adrift, making it challenging to meet our own and others' needs for support and comfort.

GIVING AND RECEIVING

These days many people are overfed but undernourished physically, mentally, and spiritually. When we overconsume instead of nourishing ourselves, our capacity to process becomes overwhelmed, and what was meant to satisfy us instead weighs us down. You can see this on both a personal and a collective level. Just like the Dampness we discussed earlier that builds up in our bodies from poor physical digestion, our fixation on consuming more and more material goods leads to Earth element congestion and eventually pathological excess on a global level. This is sadly apparent when we look at the effects of late-stage capitalism. The appeal of having "more" is strong in our modern culture and economy, and we all know how this can create enormous consumer waste and significantly increase carbon in the atmosphere. From T-shirts to toothbrushes, the machine of industrialization races to keep up with the demands of unending consumption while clogging up our beautiful planet. In turn, the earth swells as the waterways and soil attempt to manage and assimilate plastic waste and our never-ending use of resources.

On a personal level, the weaker our Earth element is, the more we contribute to this mess. With a weak Earth element, we lose touch with deeper ways to feed ourselves, we feel unsatisfied, and we look for instant gratification to comfort us instead. We seek to fill our metaphorical hunger by taking too much—consuming unhealthy foods, acquiring more stuff, or acting as if our needs are more important than those of others. As with all the elements, when Earth is out of balance, our actions further weaken us, so unhealthy craving creates unhealthy consumption, which feeds more unhealthy craving. It's a vicious cycle. It goes around and around—just like the movement of worry we looked at earlier. When this is the case, we use enormous energy to satisfy our ceaseless hunger in the pursuit of temporary satisfaction.

Addictions to food, material possessions, power, and wealth can consume us, but there are also subtler ways that craving shows up. Rather than take my word for it, consider whether there are desires (material and immaterial) that strongly sway your day-to-day activities to those that are not always good for you. Especially consider those times when you want more than you need, whether it's attention or material possessions. Daoist and Buddhist texts illustrate this phenomenon with the image of the "hungry ghosts" with tiny mouths and throats yet huge stomachs, endlessly tormented by insatiable desire, thirst, or hunger. Within the Buddhist context, this feverish thirst or craving is the primary cause of *dukkha*, or suffering. This kind of wanting is the flip side of peace; it's anchored in greed and leads to clinging and, ultimately, unhappiness. In many cases, there is nothing fundamentally wrong with the tendency to want a pleasant experience. Still, this points to something more profound: craving is a powerful state of mind that can become a strong motivating factor in our lives. If this motivation is unchecked, it can easily lead to self-centered actions and further Earth element depletion.

The Earth element develops throughout our lives and can weaken for many reasons, including protracted illness and an unhealthy diet. However, it first forms in childhood, and its health depends on our earliest experiences of being cared for physically and emotionally. Having guardians who cared for you and made you feel safe imparted an internal felt sense of security that has carried into your adult years. When I have patients like this, I recognize it because they're comfortable in their own skin; they feel deeply at home with themselves and the world. Their Earth element is strong.

On the other hand, if you didn't receive the support you needed as a child or your Earth element is weak for other reasons, you may find it difficult as an adult to harvest your life experiences, to digest the experiences you've had or find nourishment in what life offers you. When I work with these types of patients, I notice they are often overly concerned about getting their needs met or, conversely, too focused on the needs of others at the expense of their own self-care.

For instance, if your Earth element imbalance manifests as an unreasonable focus on others, you may give too much. Maybe you know someone like this: their offer of support, generosity, or concern comes with a sticky, needy, clingy vibe. Whether we offer sympathy, material help, time, or energy, when our Earth is imbalanced, we tend to get carried away. Similar to how we are inclined to overconsume when our Earth element is disordered, we can also fixate on pleasing others and being the "helper." This people-pleasing, self-sacrificing pattern is common in those involved in the helping professions. For instance, many of my students and patients who are yoga teachers, nurses, bodyworkers, and therapists have had to learn how to guard their energy levels, time, and resources—by not giving too much and prioritizing true self-care—so they're able to do their work in the world effectively. The key to healing this aspect of Earth element imbalance is staying in touch with our true intentions and nourishing our roots.

As you can see, developing the emotional and spiritual qualities of a good, stable Earth element is all about finding an equal relationship between giving and receiving and establishing a sense of internal contentment and comfort tempered with empathy, selflessness, and service. Our actions and choices matter to us and all others because a vast web of mutual codependency and co-arising links us. Thich Nhat Hanh called this "inter-being" based on the Buddha's teaching of dependent origination, namely, that all phenomena in the universe are interwoven and interdependent. We are not, in fact, isolated hungry ghosts.

Whether in our immediate family, in our neighborhood, or on a global scale, our actions ripple outward, affecting ever-widening circles of beings everywhere. When Earth element energy is balanced and secure, our thoughts, actions, and lives embody this understanding of reciprocity. We don't take too much from others or the planet, and we don't give so much that we lose contact with our own needs. Instead, we live in a place of gratitude and appreciation, giving of ourselves with empathy when we can without draining our resources. Let's explore a few practices to support us in doing that.

HEALING THE EARTH ELEMENT

> Review what you're taking in. The impressions you receive through your senses are essential in forming thoughts and, eventually, intentions and actions. Use the guidelines in Chapter 11 to fine-tune the types of foods you eat. Examine what else enters your other sense organs that you have to digest. Do you spend time and energy online? How much? What kinds of music, TV, and news do you consume? What conversations are you a part of? Are they skillful and kind? This isn't about cutting yourself off from the matters of the world. Instead, it's about being intentional about where you put your focus and for how long.

> Clear your thoughts. If you pay attention, you'll probably notice you're filled with all kinds of undigested gristle, especially if you get caught up in excessive rumination. Take some time to sift through the disarray. One way to do this is with journaling. Carve out some time to release your thoughts onto paper. Especially if you've had a big life event recently, give yourself time to digest it like a large meal. If you find yourself spinning out in worry, focus on one concern and make an action plan. What is one small step you can take today to move forward with this issue? You can also organize your thoughts regularly with a to-do list. Return to your list as you take action and complete tasks. Then, when the inclination arises to mull that thought or worry over again, remind yourself you already wrote it down. It's on your list, and you'll attend to it when you can.

> Focus on self-care and inner contentment (*santosha*). The Earth element flourishes fully when we know how to self-soothe and regularly take care of ourselves. This kind of self-care is not

elaborate. It simply means focusing on all your basic needs and practicing not always needing more. Rather than waiting until you are overextended or exhausted, make sure you are eating well, exercising, and getting good sleep every day. Also, routinely enjoy a few uncomplicated experiences that you find personally satisfying, like playing a game, taking a bath, being in nature, or spending time with a pet.

> Tend to your home nest. Our sense of home is a big focus for the Earth element. If your space feels too full, get rid of what you no longer need. Clean the clutter and create a warm, welcoming, comfortable, and safe place. Reflect on how you can nurture this feeling of home wherever you are. You could also do research into the history of where you live. Unless you are native to the land you live on, consider how you might acknowledge the many generations of Indigenous people before you who cared for and lived in the place you now call home. To create even deeper roots, you can also extend this inquiry to include the plants and animals you share the space with.

> Practice gratitude and receiving. Make a habit of pausing and giving thanks on a regular basis. This could be when you experience something you appreciate like a delicious meal or when someone does something for you or offers a kind word. Consciously receive the gifts life gives you and savor them.

Clarifying Your Intentions

Clear intentions that we consistently act on are one of the fruits we harvest from a healthy Earth element. Intentions are similar to goals, but they have essential differences. Goals are future-oriented and usually designed to achieve a particular result. Intentions, on the other hand, help you find the reasons behind your goals and ensure you act based on your deeper values.

For this contemplation, we'll do some journaling. Begin by finding a comfortable place where you feel relaxed, present, and available. To begin, write freely as you consider your intentions. What is it that motivates you? As you reflect, you may observe your surface conditioning—the part of you that craves or rejects. For instance, you may want that job, that relationship, or some other object or accomplishment. Take some time to explore the deeper meaning of your desires. If you achieved those goals, how would it make you feel? How would your life experience be different?

Next, ponder your deepest values. What is most important to you? It could be qualities like patience, equality, or kindness toward yourself and others. Genuine intentions, as they relate to the spirit of the Earth element, are rooted in care and generosity toward all beings. Now reflect on your daily habits and regular actions. Do they align with your intentions and values? If not, why not? Try not to judge. Instead, stay open, loving, and curious.

Once you have established your deeper motives, you can focus on or state your intention. Try writing it down or saying it out loud or silently to yourself. Try using the present tense or the introductory phrase "May I be," which helps you connect with your longing and embody your intended state. You could say something like, "May I be kind," "May I be compassionate," or "May I be patient." Creating an intentional vow is a profound recognition that the quality you seek already exists within and is immediately accessible.

Last, remember there is a contradiction inherent in the practice of intention. I learned this once from the meditation teacher Phillip Moffitt, and I've found it helpful. At any given time, you have the opportunity to "be" your intention, and at the same time, you're constantly "becoming" it. As you move through life, you will inevitably notice that you haven't fully embodied your intentions, especially under challenging circumstances or when you become overly fixated on your goals. When you recognize you're not acting from your deeper intentions, you can always return to the simplicity of your vow: "May I be kind. . . ." This return repeatedly reminds you of your deeper motives and can act as a center point to guide the compass of your life. When you connect with your intentions, you ultimately gain access to your true nature and your Dao. Your Dao exists within you, guided by your heart's longing, and you can feel it and hear it if you tune in and listen.

Sama Vritti Pranayama (Equal Breathing)

———

In this practice, we even out the breath, making the inhalation and exhalation the same length. Because the Earth element is all about stabilizing our center and this breath is about creating evenness, it is particularly helpful to harmonize Earth element energies.

Using a folded blanket or cushion, find an upright seated posture supporting your pelvis with a 4- to 6-inch lift. Relax your body and place your hands on your legs or lap. Use the first few minutes of this practice to get in touch with your breath and simply notice how it is right now. Once you are relatively calm and present, continue with the guidelines that follow.

In the first stage of pranayama, we regulate the breath to become smooth and slow. As you relax and pay attention to your breathing, you may notice that it has naturally slowed down of its own accord. I once heard this process described as calming a frightened bird. Slowly and with patience, the wings of the breath settle and become tranquil. This easy and unhurried breathing enlivens every cell and tissue in the body and brings more clarity and space to the mind.

Once this is accomplished and easily maintained, the next step is to lengthen the breath gently. Slowly and gradually, encourage the breath to elongate slightly, either when you inhale, when you exhale, or both. Never force the breath to change; instead, endeavor to create a relationship with the breath in which warmth and trust can develop over time. Continue with this practice if you want, simply using the remainder of your time to slow and slightly lengthen the breath.

If you choose to carry on, we'll create Sama Vritti— an evening out of the breath—by creating an equal inhalation to exhalation ratio. Start by determining what your natural breath count is right now. For example, through observation and counting, you may discover that you inhale to a count of six and exhale to a count of seven. For Sama Vritti, aim to inhale and exhale for the same amount of time. You can do this in several ways: increasing the shorter count, shortening the longer count, or meeting somewhere in the middle. Try all three methods and see if you prefer one. Finally, if you find the counting intrusive and distracting, you can also do this practice by simply sensing into the lengths of breath and evening them that way. In any case, continue to practice for 10 to 15 minutes.

Walking Meditation

When I first started exploring walking meditations on longer silent retreats, I was surprised to discover that the movement of walking relieved the sleepiness and aches and pains I was experiencing from long sitting meditation periods. In fact, walking meditation soon became the place where I could drop into very deep states of concentration and awareness. If you give walking meditation a try, you may be delighted to discover it has some unique and striking effects because of the way walking moves Qi and connects you to earth.

The formal way of practicing walking meditation involves choosing a small area in which to walk back and forth. I invite you to expand that a bit and find somewhere you can walk in nature, so you can more fully connect to the earth and natural elements. Remember, you're not walking to get anywhere! There is no destination. Your focus is on the walking itself, which gives you an opportunity to build embodied presence while doing something you probably most often do unconsciously.

To begin, choose a place where you can walk with ease; it should be about 30 feet or so. To practice, you'll walk to the end of your path, pause, turn around and walk back; over and over again until your meditation period concludes. Practice the Grounding Stance (from Chapter 11) for 5 to 10 minutes first; that will enhance your presence and your connection to the earth before you walk.

As you begin walking, find a pace that works for you. Stay connected to your breath and the sensations and feelings in your body. Some people find this slows their pace considerably, others find they like to walk a little quicker. Choose a speed that feels relaxed and allows you to stay present in your body. Experiment with feeling your whole body or zoom into one aspect, like the gradual pressure of each foot as it lands on the ground. The more intimately connected to the movement you become, the more likely you are to feel and sense how your gait echoes throughout the muscles and bones of your entire body or how the many small and intricate movements in your foot and ankle all cooperate to take one step.

As you walk, remain soft and receptive. If something in your environment strikes you, you can stop and notice it—take in the sights, colors, sounds, and smells around you. Then continue walking, refocusing your mind on the task at hand in a gentle yet concentrated way. Practice for 15 to 30 minutes.

The Earth element holds special importance because it sustains and benefits all other elements. We've examined how its capacity to digest and assimilate manifests in nature and our bodies and minds. When balanced, Earth's qualities are nurturing and stable. In the Five Element cycle, Earth generates Metal. In our next section we'll explore the season of the Metal element—one of clearing and deceleration.

AUTUMN SEASON & METAL ELEMENT

THIRTEEN

AUTUMN SLOWING & THE METAL ELEMENT

Another world is not only possible, she's on her way. Maybe many of us won't be here to greet her, but on a quiet day, if I listen very carefully, I can hear her breathing.[37]
—ARUNDHATI ROY

Each of us is a tiny speck in the universe imbued with and connected to the cosmos through the Metal element. Earth's metals began billions of years ago with the dawn of the universe and the explosion of stars and asteroids. After these original collisions, metals traveled to Earth as gas and dust. Metals that form planet Earth (and our human bodies) are literally created from stardust. From the Daoist perspective, the Metal element symbolizes mountains and all metals like gold and silver, minerals, and precious gems. Today, metals are spread throughout the earth's layers and crust and are mixed with rocks and minerals to form ore. Certain metals, such as copper, magnesium, zinc, and iron, are essential to life and are found in nearly all living matter in the form of minerals and trace minerals. For example, iron is found in hemoglobin, a crucial component of human blood. Chlorophyll, necessary for photosynthesis and plant life, contains magnesium. Without these necessary metals, life would cease to exist. In many ways, Metal is the most hidden of the elements. Like underground caves full of gleaming gems and gold, Metal is not always visible, but it's still present under the cloak of Earth and circulating within our bodies. In Chinese medicine, the Metal element in our bodies and minds requires both taking in and letting go. It is responsible for the precious air we breathe and the waste we release. On a psychospiritual level, it exemplifies the idea that we are spiritual beings in physical bodies. It teaches us that our human life is about finding value and inspiration and coming to terms with loss and mortality.

In the Five Element model, Metal is a contractive declining energy. The transition to this element is one of declining Yang and increasing Yin. When we look at the natural world, we see this decline most clearly in the slowing and rooting time of autumn. Autumn is a time of loss; a season of pulling back and allowing things to draw naturally to a close. It represents completion and a descent into the underworld. The *Nei Jing* states, "The three months of autumn, they denote taking in and balance. The qi of heaven becomes tense. The qi of earth becomes bright . . . it is the Way to nourish gathering."[38]

As the light wanes and the days become shorter and darker, much of the natural world prepares to migrate or hibernate. Leaves dwindle, the winter squash gets picked off the vines, and the calendula goes to seed. Where I live, early autumn echoes with the steady calls of migrating Canada geese forming a perfect V across a crisp blue sky. Somber shades of gray and an ethereal tone that is almost translucent gradually sweep the landscape. Plants draw their sap inward and dive into the ground, their deep roots growing stronger, seeking nourishment from the mineral-rich soil below. Aboveground, shadows grow long; the warm smell of woodsmoke lingers in the valley; and a shroud of cool air and mist signals a season of death, decay, and interiority. It is a time to pare down. In the forest beyond my home, the northern flickers and blue jays pick off the last red berries from the mountain ash, and black bears ready their fat reserves, while squirrels, mice, and beavers gather supplies for the long winter ahead. It's a time of hunkering down, of coming home to ourselves and to what is most important.

The Metal season of autumn is considered a threshold in many traditions, when the veil to the otherworld is thin enough to contact ancestral spirits. Autumnal leaves releasing their final hold remind us of our mortality; this season offers a pause to consider past lessons and a time to honor the dead. In many traditions, the ghosts of the dead return home and must be appeased during this season. This time of year also marks the ancient holy day of Samhain in the pagan calendar. Pagans celebrate Samhain as a time when the boundaries between the living and spirit world dissipate, and one can access subtler energies ordinarily obscured. Ancestor worship is found in many diverse cultures worldwide and is one of the earth's oldest religious rites. For example, in Mexico and across Latin America, Dia de Los Muertos (Day of the Dead) is celebrated at this time with elaborate decorations and altars paying homage to those who have passed. These festivities date back to the Mayans and Aztecs, many decades before Spanish colonization. In India and worldwide, Hindus honor their ancestors during Pitru Paksha, a sixteen-day period that usually lands near the autumn equinox. Various traditions worldwide honor kin with special food offerings throughout late summer and autumn. Today in the West, this season is most often associated with the Christian event All Saints Day or the celebration of All Hallows Eve (Halloween).

Honoring death can teach us powerful lessons. During the late autumn, the trees losing their leaves poignantly show us that letting go is a natural part of existence. The trees don't die; they simply draw their energy inward in preparation for a period of growth when their inner resources become more important than their external expression. We, too, need time to strip away and turn inward. Like the autumn squash, everything ripens and decays in time. Death is not the opposite of life; it is a required *part* of life. In the great wheel of time, death is the opposite of birth. Within the Five Element cycle, the Metal element symbolizes how maturation and eventual degeneration are necessary. Without it, we wouldn't experience the potency of winter and the Water element or the light of spring and the visionary capacity of the Wood element. The minerals and nutrients of the fallen leaves will feed next year's growth, and our ability to release what no longer serves us creates space for something new to emerge. Savvy gardeners know that intelligently pruning and weeding support healthy growth. Metal represents the space available after dissolution, the elegance created through letting go or simplifying.

On a metaphysical level, many Metal element qualities are closely related to the rarefied Space or Ether (*Akasha*) element in Ayurvedic medicine. The defining characteristics of Space, according to Ayurveda, are mainly based on the absence of certain qualities rather than their presence. For example, Space is considered cold in Ayurveda because it lacks Fire, which is warm. It is light because of the absence of Earth and Water, which are stable and heavy. Similarly, in Chinese medicine, the Metal element implies spaciousness. Just as the fields lay fallow and empty in autumn, Metal represents a special liminal zone where we can access the intangible, the spiritual, the supernatural, the heavenly, or the esoteric. This space is a place of subtlety and spirit. The French composer Claude Debussy once said that "music is the space between the notes," pointing to the beauty and potential of the untouched openness between known and tangible things. During classes, I sometimes direct students to observe the expanse and moment of emptiness between breaths or thoughts to touch this quality. When we let go and attune to the awe of Space, we're more able to breathe, connect with presence, and are more likely to notice what is most meaningful and attend to it.

The Chinese character for this element shows a covering protecting flecks of precious stones or minerals in the earth below. Metal portrays what is most treasured; it represents the glint of rare deposits in stone and the hidden inner core or golden nugget of your true nature. The reflective crystalline surface of precious gems reminds us of the value and clarity we carry inside. Like the determined miner chipping away at rock to uncover its rare deposits, we must eliminate the excess and cut out whatever gets in the way of unearthing our deep and abiding intrinsic value. Pema Chödrön says, "Only to the extent that we expose ourselves over and over to annihilation can that which is indestructible be found in us."[39] Letting go of the extraneous can highlight our priorities and answer important questions, such as "What is essential and cherished?" Our central task during the Metal phase is to eliminate what is unnecessary and preserve what is priceless. As we trim back the superfluous and appreciate what is crucial, we find and illuminate what was here all along—the reflective, timeless jewel of open, spacious awareness.

METAL IMAGERY AND LANGUAGE

A sharp knife

A shield

Open sky

An exhalation and last breath

Animal instincts

Leaves falling

A dark, misty forest

A crystal-laden cave

Ghosts and spirits

Sunset

Mushrooms growing on a decaying log

Witches and the occult

Alchemy

Stone monuments

Panning for gold

Space exploration

A snake shedding its skin

ENERGETICS OF METAL CHART

Season	Autumn
Yin organ	Lung
Yang organ	Large Intestine
Tissue	Skin
Sense organ	Nose
Emotion	Grief
Direction	Downward
Sound	Crying
Climatic influence	Dryness
Taste	Pungent
Color	White

SEASONAL SELF-CARE FOR AUTUMN

In autumn we focus, gather, and simplify. You might notice a feeling of homecoming during this season—this is a time when you can settle in and slow down a bit. Autumn encourages us to tap into what is greater than us, hold close what is precious, and release what has passed. Here are some ways to harmonize with the slowing and rooting season.

> Consider how your body or mind may need a release and do some housekeeping. Ask yourself, "Are there ways of thinking or being I'm ready to let go? Has something been maturing that is ready to be released? Are there relationships or physical possessions I no longer value that I want to relinquish?"

> Spend more time at home and slow down by saying no when you can to engagements that are not authentic or truly valuable to you.

> Focus on spiritual practice and try early morning meditation, contemplation, or prayer. The early morning, right before and just after sunrise, is connected to the Metal element in TCM and is called *brahmamuhurta* in Ayurveda, meaning "sacred time" or "time of Brahma." You may remember that Brahma means "ultimate reality," which is similar to the concept of Dao. This time is especially auspicious and precious, making it the best time for spiritual practice, especially in autumn.

> Incorporate more grounding practices into your daily routine, such as longer-held standing and balance poses, to counteract the scattered and hectic feeling often present in autumn.

> Monitor your energy levels carefully. Rest and nap when you need to.

> Stay warm as temperatures drop. Wear extra layers and take hot baths.

> Make sure you are having regular bowel movements. In autumn, Dryness may cause constipation. Energetically, the most beneficial time for a bowel movement is in the morning between 5 A.M. and 7 A.M. Drink warm water as soon as you get up, and eat enough fiber in the form of cooked fresh vegetables, whole grains,

seeds, beans, and legumes to help. Try stewing apples with prunes in a little water to support healthy elimination during this season.

> If you have sinus congestion, seasonal allergies, or trouble breathing, or if you tend to get sick this time of year, try using *neti* and *nasya* (an Ayurvedic practice of rinsing the nasal passages with warm, purified saltwater and oiling the nose).

> Massage natural oils into your body to support your skin and lymph channels and create a natural barrier between you and the outer elements. Read more about this practice in Chapter 14.

AUTUMN KITCHEN MEDICINE

In autumn, temperatures cool, and the crisp winds have a bite. Now is the time to prepare the body for winter. In Ayurveda, *vata* dosha, which has cold, dry, and mobile qualities, increases. In TCM, we also protect against Dryness and Cold. It's a great time to build up our tissues and store energy for the coming months.

In autumn aim to eat nourishing, heartier foods that provide moisture. Stay away from excessively spicy or frozen options, and instead choose cooked, naturally sweet, and protein-rich foods. If you're feeling dry and cold as winter approaches, focus on supplementing your Yin and warming your body with healthy oils and meals with extra liquid, such as soups and stews. Follow these recommendations during autumn for health all season long:

> It's okay to eat more this time of year. Follow your appetite and enjoy heavier meals if needed.

> Aim to nourish the deep tissues of your body with whole grains, nuts, seeds, eggs, lentils, and small dark beans such as adzuki.

> Add more cooked foods to your diet, and try cooking in ways that concentrate flavor, such as for longer periods of time at lower temperatures.

> If the weather is cold or damp, add warming and aromatic spices and foods like cloves, cinnamon, garlic, ginger, and onions.

> Drink warm water and herbal teas throughout the day.

> Add foods that have naturally sweet flavors, like root vegetables. Try carrots, parsnips, sweet potatoes, beets, and winter squash.
> Eat moistening foods and healthy oils like soy milk, tofu, seaweed, avocado, spiced dairy, oats, pears, tahini, olive oil, ghee, and sesame oil.
> Use small amounts of salty and sour flavors. Try sauerkraut, sourdough bread, yogurt, olives, pickles, and rose hip tea.
> Avoid dry foods like crackers and chips; reduce raw and cold foods.
> Herbal medicines at this time of year should focus on supporting your respiratory system, healthy elimination, and immunity. Use herbs like cordyceps (*dong chong xia cao*) and echinacea. My favorite classical formula for this season is Jade Windscreen (*Yu Ping Feng San*). This formula's name suggests that it creates a "screen from the wind" that is precious and strong, like jade. It is helpful if you get sick easily, are prone to seasonal allergies, or feel like you might be getting a common cold.

As you can see, the resonance of the Metal element helps us strip everything back to what is purest and most essential. We can work with this energy by observing its presence in nature and through seasonal food and self-care choices. However, the Metal element also lives within us—its expression can be seen in our organs and our subtle energetic system, which we explore here, and in our emotions and spiritual life, which we'll examine in the next two chapters.

ORGANS OF THE METAL ELEMENT

In Chinese medicine, the organs associated with Metal are the Lungs, which include the entire respiratory passageway—the nose, nasal passages, and trachea—and the Large Intestine. Physically, the lungs are located in the chest on either side of the heart above the diaphragm. They are essential respiratory organs in the human body, exchanging oxygen and carbon dioxide between the air we breathe and our bloodstream. The large intestine is the final part of the long and winding gastrointestinal tract. As food and fluid move through the digestive tract, the large intestine completes the process by absorbing water and storing and excreting waste. It is also responsible for housing gut bacteria that produce specific vitamins.

In Chinese medicine, the Lung and Large Intestine also have energetic functions (in TCM, this organ is not plural, we call it "the Lung"). The Large Intestine has a similar function to its Western counterpart of reabsorbing fluids and eliminating waste, but it also has a unique relationship with the Lung in that they work together harmoniously to ensure that Qi descends when it needs to. For instance, if your Large Intestine is not eliminating waste adequately, causing constipation, you may experience a worsening of allergy or breathing symptoms. In TCM, the Lung governs Qi and respiration; it facilitates the free circulation and diffusion of Qi and Body Fluids in all channels and the space between the skin and muscles, as well as regulating water passages. Because the Lung has such a close relationship to Qi through its function of breathing in and circulating Qi, it also regulates all physiological activities in the body. Therefore, if I have a patient showing signs of low vitality or any breathing concerns—for instance, chronic obstructive pulmonary disease, shortness of breath, asthma, a weak voice, pale skin, fatigue, or excessive weight loss—I'll assess whether their Lung Qi provides adequate energy. The Lung is also responsible for the health of the nose, throat, and nasal passages, so concerns such as recurrent infections there or a loss of sense of smell are also an indication of imbalance.

The Lung is the most sensitive organ because it acts as our first barrier to outside influences, along with the skin and respiratory passages. In particular, it circulates a special kind of Qi called Wei Qi. Think of the Wei Qi as an energetic shield that lies near the body's surface, outside the main meridians and between the skin and muscles. It warms and protects the body from external attackers by mixing with sweat and regulating the opening and closing of the pores. Like the Western understanding of immunity and the lymphatic system, the Wei Qi mounts a defense. If an outside pathogen is stronger than our defense, it may overpower this protective barrier and we get sick. This can happen if we're exposed to a common cold or environmental pathogen, for example, or if we get a chill. When the Wei and Lung Qi are weak, the body is more susceptible to illness. If this system is not healthy, you might have a weak immune system, catch colds frequently, or have acute skin issues from outside influences like seasonal rashes or allergies.

The body's exterior—especially body hair, skin, and sweat glands—are related to Lung Qi, so imbalances commonly present as chronic skin conditions such as eczema or dryness. It is interesting to note that TCM links the health of the skin to both breathing and the function of the Large Intestine. In my clinical practice, I find it common for patients with food sensitivities that lead to constipation and malabsorption to have also had a long history of childhood asthma and eczema. In such cases, we usually work to eliminate food triggers, reestablish good digestion, and treat any imbalance in the Metal element and immune system.

METAL ELEMENT MERIDIANS

The Sinew channels of the Lung travel from the palm side of the thumbs, up the inner arms to the chest, ribs, and diaphragm. The Large Intestine's Sinew channels begin at the tips of the index fingers and ascend the outer arms to the lateral side of the elbows; they then travel up to the shoulders, neck, face, and top of the head with branches to the shoulder blades and thoracic spine. Postures that lengthen, compress, open, squeeze, and apply pressure to these target areas can be helpful for harmonizing the Metal element and the flow of Qi through its subtle body channels.

To support these channels and subtler meridians associated with the energetic Lung and Large Intestine, and the Metal element in general, we can choose specific movements and yoga postures that target the tissues in the arms, upper back, chest, diaphragm, and lower abdomen. When the Metal element is imbalanced, it is common for students to experience congestion in the colon, which can hinder their breathing. In yoga this indicates an imbalance between *prana vayu*—an energetic wind related to breathing—and *apana vayu*—a downward wind connected to elimination. Movements that alternately compress and release these areas will be beneficial in harmonizing the movement of energy and reestablishing balance.

Sensing and Compressing the Metal Element Channels and Organs

Lie flat on your back on a firm but soft surface, like a blanket spread over a yoga mat. Exhale deeply a few times and allow your body to drop and release. As you relax, invite your breath to slow and deepen. Notice if you seem to be holding yourself up from the ground. Bring your attention to your lower abdomen, respiratory diaphragm, and chest.

The powerful respiratory diaphragm is a significant muscle involved with breathing and disseminating Qi throughout the body, making it a Metal element structure. All fascial structures move in tandem with the diaphragm, so working with this structure is essential to whole-body health. Shaped like a dome covering a large area, it connects many structures of the torso, including the ribs, internal organs of the abdomen, and lumbar spine, through a pliable myofascial network. Hence, tension in this structure can translate into not only breathing difficulties but many other concerns like hip and back pain, pelvic floor dysfunction, and even digestion issues like constipation. As you lie on your back, allow your diaphragm to widen and soften. Don't force; use time and space to slowly relax.

Now bring your attention to your shoulders. Do they seem to fall forward toward your chest (lift off the floor)? Begin to visualize the energetic pathway of the Lung channel along your inner arms and the Large Intestine channel along your outer arms. Feel one side of your body and then the other. Is one side more tense or lax? Scan your arms and upper chest; notice if your fingers curl more into one palm than the other or if you feel any other tugging or sensation. Quietly observe what somatic pattern is showing up in your body.

Next, bring your awareness to your physical lungs and large intestine. Your rectum, near the end of your large intestine, attaches to your pelvic floor at the base of your trunk. Invite your pelvic floor to soften and the large intestine above it to relax downward. Feel or imagine your lungs filling the space of your chest. The tissues of your lungs grow directly into your diaphragm. As your diaphragm moves up and down with breathing, the membranes of your chest move along with it. All of these structures are designed to work cooperatively with one another, however they go out of sync and become stifled when imbalanced.

Shining white is the color we associate with these organs. If it helps, you can place your hands on your lower abdomen and upper chest for a moment. As you breathe, imagine a bright white light infusing your energetic Lung and Large Intestine with energy. Stay visualizing this color for 5 to 10 breaths. To exit the pose, relax any focus and roll to one side.

Next, we'll use a rolled blanket to create mild pressure on the malleable structures of the upper and lower abdomen where the connections in and around the diaphragm converge and the physical large intestine lies.

Place a soft rolled blanket crosswise on your mat. Lay your belly on the roll so the blanket is putting gentle pressure on your upper abdomen just below your lower ribs. Do not put direct pressure on the xiphoid process (the bony bit below the sternum or breastbone). Find a position where you feel some pressure on the tissues but nothing painful. Control the pressure by using your forearms and elbows. Start with a few slow, controlled pumping movements. Release your elbows, allowing more pressure on your belly from the blanket, then ease up a little by pressing your arms into the floor, lessening the pressure of the torso on the blanket. After a few times, pause in a place that feels good and concentrate on some long, slow breaths into the area where you feel the blanket's pressure. Don't force the breath; instead, feel the tactile feedback of the blanket as you breathe. After a few breath cycles, you can adjust the blanket to a slightly different position (lower or higher, depending on where you started) and try again. Once you've finished, push yourself up.

Come into kneeling, sitting back on your heels. If possible, bring your knees close together. This time, place your blanket roll on your lap. Tuck it right up against your belly so it is snuggled against your hips and abdomen. Press the blanket down into your legs and lift your belly. Now fold forward into Child's Pose. If your head doesn't meet the floor, use a prop like a blanket or yoga block under your forehead. As with the first blanket roll, find a position that feels comfortable, not painful. Aim for a slightly stronger sensation—you can make the roll bigger or smaller, depending on your preference. Relax and take some long, slow breaths into the lower abdominal area where you feel the blanket's pressure. Don't force it; simply feel the pressure of the blanket as you breathe.

To conclude the practice, sit up, remove the prop, and lie on your back for a few breaths, feeling any new sense of space in the abdomen and diaphragm.

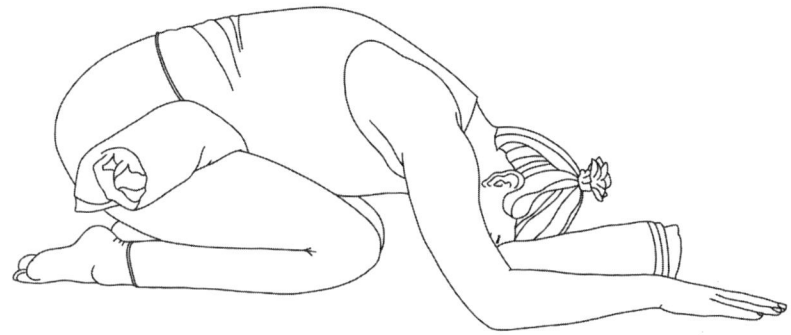

FOURTEEN

BREATHING SPACE

The True One breathes from the heels;
ordinary people breathe from their throats.[40]
—CHUANG TZU

The conclusive song of Metal is one of release and letting go. However, its resonance is also one of precious value, purity and clarity. We've explored how these qualities are manifest in nature and in our bodies. Now we can look at how they might go out of balance and practices to help.

METAL ELEMENT BREATHING

When it comes to Metal element health, one of the primary ways imbalance occurs is through disordered breathing. Your breathing reflects the deep patterns held in your psyche and soma, and it's at the center of your energetic health. When your breathing is dysfunctional, your body-mind doesn't get the oxygen and Qi it needs, and everything suffers.

Breathing, of course, is the movement that happens during respiration and is essential for human life. The moment you are born, you inhale your first breath; the moment you leave this world, you exhale your last. It's easy to view breathing in such a limited way. Yes, it affects the lungs and exchanges oxygen and carbon dioxide in the body, but it's so much more than that. The ever-moving breath is our steady companion and a powerful access point into the subtle body. Did you know the word *breath* means "spirit," "soul," or "life force" in many languages? The Chinese symbol for Qi translates as "breath," and the same word is used in Latin for both breath and spirit! Through respiration, the Daoists say we take in the "Qi of heaven," receiving fresh inspiration and energy in the shape of an enlivening and dynamic force.

In the Ayurvedic and yogic systems, this correlates with the concept of Prana, which is the breath *and* the fundamental life force circulating through our system. The Sanskrit word *prana* comes from the root *an*, similar to the word for sentient being (*pranaka*), signifying that without breath, there is no life. Essentially, the diaphragm's movement initiates the flow of this life force into every organ, tissue, nerve, and fluid. In Chinese medicine, the breath combines with the energy we receive from food to comprise *Zong* (gathering) Qi, which collects in the chest in an area called the "Sea of Qi." Zong Qi supports the Lung and Heart by circulating Blood and Qi to the rest of the body—especially to our limbs and hands. It also supports a strong voice. If I have a patient with poor circulation in their hands, a feeble voice, or weak or shallow breathing, I assess how this function is working. The various practices of lengthening, controlling, and restraining the breath (called pranayama in yoga) aim to increase and conserve this vital life force.

I probably don't have to tell you all the amazing ways breathing affects us. It impacts respiratory, immune, nervous, and hormonal systems. It alters digestion, moods, energy levels, and sleep. The breath can cause us to explode in reactive behavior or help us remain calm and centered under pressure. Even so, we spend most of our time unaware of the body's breathing. One reason is that the continual stream of breath blends effortlessly with other actions and movements. It remains constant whether we're sleeping, singing, jogging, or snacking. However, breathing is not just automatic; it is one of the few bodily functions that is both automatic *and* voluntary. It is an automatic exchange between your internal and external environment, and you can directly affect it. With this in mind, the breath is an excellent teacher. It can show us when we're holding too tightly and not letting go; when we're collapsed and not allowing new inspiration and energy in; and when we're feeling inspired, safe, spacious, and energized.

It is important to note that healthy breathing is not simply about how deeply we breathe or how much breath we take in. Rather it is the quality and efficiency of the breath that counts. Our breath can become dysfunctional for many reasons and in many ways. A good place to start discovering your pattern of disharmony is through simple awareness. When you breathe, are you at ease, as if you're moving in the same direction as a meandering stream, or are you rushed, tense, or forceful, moving against the tide? Healthy breathing increases vitality like nothing else because it directly supplies the body-mind with oxygen, Qi, and greater Blood flow and supports healthy Wei Qi—the protective barrier on the surface of your body related to immunity. Learning to work with and regulate your breathing supports your nervous system; can calm your mind and prepare you for internal practices like meditation; and creates greater movement in your diaphragm, which stimulates many internal organs. We'll cover some breathing practices in this chapter and the next.

Habits for Healthy Breathing

If you want to strengthen your Metal element and support healthy breathing, here are a few habits to implement right away:

> First, find your breath. The first stage in developing healthy breathing patterns is to notice how it moves naturally without manipulation. I call this uncovering your breath. This practice doesn't always come easily! Chances are, if you've been practicing yoga for any length of time, you've already learned many ways to *change* your breathing for specific practices. Many people have unconscious and disordered breathing habits. If you jump immediately into changing the breath without first discovering your holding, numbing, or tensing patterns, you risk layering breathing practices onto a faulty foundation. Start with a regular practice of simply noticing your breath. Pause throughout your day and ask yourself, "How does my breath feel? Where do I notice it in my body? Is my breath fast or slow? Am I holding my breath right now?" As you work with this practice, you will notice that

your awareness and observations become subtler. Paying attention to the breath automatically changes it as it shifts your Qi away from external demands and toward your body. Take note of how your breathing pattern changes from day to day. Especially as you work with the practices in this book, you may notice your breath becoming more graceful and relaxed with time.

> Breathe through your nose. The nose is the sense organ we most closely associate with the Metal element as it's essential for breathing. It contains mucous membranes and tiny hairs that protect your respiratory passageway from harmful particles, pollutants, and germs. It warms and moistens the air, preparing it to go deeper into your body. Nasal breathing also supports meditative awareness. If you have a condition that makes nasal breathing impossible, you can breathe with your mouth or a combination of your nose and mouth.

> Develop natural breathing. The most life-giving and efficient way to breathe is through natural diaphragmatic breathing, which means the respiratory diaphragm moves down and the abdomen expands on inhalation. On exhalation, the diaphragm moves up and the abdomen contracts. This kind of breath is not forceful and does not involve tensing. Instead, it requires relaxation. During natural breathing, the breath changes according to activity levels. For instance, during aerobic activity, your breathing will become more apparent, faster, and deeper; during quiet reflection, it may become small and soft. However, at all times, the primary movement of a natural and healthy breath happens in the abdomen due to the movement of the diaphragm, even if it's barely perceptible. Focus on gently addressing possible hindrances to the natural expression of your breath by softening areas of tension and allowing your diaphragm to relax. If you notice that your breath is limited by tension in your belly or chest, can you consciously relax? Once you feel your breath is more flexible and fully integrated and you're able to easily maintain this experience, you can move on to changing the breath for specific aims, as in the practices later in this chapter.

OUR SENSITIVE BARRIER

In the same way that the Metal element connects us to our first line of defense—our Lung, nose, respiratory passageways, and Wei Qi—it is also connected to our skin.

The skin is the largest organ in the body and manages a significant range of responsibilities. It helps regulate temperature, participates in your immune system through a vast network of lymph vessels, excretes waste through sweat glands, and is involved in metabolism, among other functions. In Chinese medical diagnosis, the state of the skin—including any abnormal marks, luster, and color—indicates the health of our Lung Qi, the overall state of our Qi and Blood, and how well our organs work together. In addition, our skin often reflects other imbalances with symptoms like rashes, eczema, and acne. In the last chapter, we covered how the Wei Qi, governed by the energetic Lung, circulates just beneath the skin, protecting us from external pathogens. The skin also acts as one of our primary sense doors. It receives sensory impressions from the environment and relays this information to the central nervous system. As a sensitive barrier, the skin provides a framework for us to know the world and our place in it. It effectively defines what is "us" and what is "not us." The skin helps us understand our surroundings and determine who we are at a very primal level. One who feels "at home in their skin" has a good sense of self in relation to the world.

One way to support your skin is through the nourishing practice of *abhyanga*, or Ayurvedic oil massage. I find this practice is unparalleled in healing the Metal element because it encourages somatic connection, which is the spiritual quality of the Metal element we'll explore in the next chapter. Abhyanga helps to rid the body of wastes, slow aging, nourish the skin, increase lymphatic flow, and support healthy immunity by protecting and preserving the Wei Qi you learned about earlier.

Abhyanga

In abhyanga, we massage warm, sometimes medicated, oil into the body. This practice helps to bolster the body's tissues and support the nervous system, and it can be especially healing if you're feeling exhausted and depleted. Abhyanga is especially helpful during the Metal element season of autumn because it counteracts Cold and Dryness and qualities like roughness and mobility associated with vata in Ayurveda—that increase during the fall. It can also be helpful if you travel a lot or don't have a regular routine because it relieves the Yin-depleting, erratic, and light qualities that can become exaggerated during travel and excessive activity.

Use abhyanga in the morning to help with detoxification or in the evening to aid sleep and support relaxation. The frequency will depend on your stress levels, age, and season—and how depleted you are. If you can't practice it daily, begin with using it once a week. Avoid abhyanga right after eating, when you have an acute cold or mucous congestion, during hot and damp weather, during menstruation, or when you have symptoms of dampness or ama (a sticky, toxic residue primarily from poor digestion; refer to Chapter 11 to learn more about digestive stagnation). Finally, using a lot of oil can get messy! Remember to designate a few towels you don't mind getting oily, and clean your bathtub regularly to avoid clogging the drain and having slippery accidents.

To begin this practice, first pick your oil. Use only *natural refined oil* (organic, if possible), not lotion. Do not use mineral oil or oils with synthetic scents or colors. The type of oil is usually chosen based on your constitution or imbalance. If you're unsure which type to choose, start with a neutral oil like almond; if you feel cold or live in a cold climate, you can try a warming oil like sesame; coconut oil is nice if you lean toward feeling hot or live in a hot environment.

Set yourself up in a warm bathroom by laying out an old towel (it will get oily). For this practice, warm the oil; room temperature or cold oil will clog the energetic channels and won't have the intended effect. Warm the oil using a double boiler–type arrangement; put the oil in a small jar or container, and place that container in a pot with a bit of water to heat it. Once the oil is warm, you're ready for your massage. Remove your clothes, and slowly work a generous amount of oil into your body, completely covering all the curves and crevices, focusing on those places that feel tender or need a little extra attention.

Start by massaging the oil into your face, ears, nose, and neck. Make long, sweeping movements on your arms and legs and circular movements around your joints like the shoulders, elbows, and knees. Slow down and check in with yourself. How does your body feel today? Move to your chest, abdomen, back, and sides. Don't forget your feet and hands too! It should take around 10 minutes to do your entire body.

Once you have finished, sit back and relax, letting the oil sink in for another 5 to 10 minutes. The longer you allow the oil to absorb, the more benefit you will experience. Once you have rested, step into the shower or a hot bath and use soap only in the places where you need it. Bathing without soap *after* the oil massage will encourage the oil to sink in more deeply. When you get out of the shower, pat yourself dry. Then move through the rest of your day with greater grounding and a deep sense of nourishment.

PRACTICES FOR BALANCE

To work with the Metal element system in movement and meditation, use practices that bring attention inward and focus on subtle sensation and somatic awareness. Breathing practices, such as pranayama, and movements that encourage flexibility and flow in the lungs, diaphragm, arms, shoulders, upper back, side body, and colon free up the movement of Qi to circulate, restoring vital energy. Shoulder openers, arm balances, twists, inversions, supported and unsupported backbends, and side bends all work well.

Somatic Side Bending with Palace of Heaven

This movement involves a flowing, side-bending, somatic motion combined with a longer-held side-bending pose I've found particularly helpful in opening restricted breathing.

To begin, lie on your back on a firm but soft surface, like a blanket spread over a yoga mat. Place your elbows on the floor and your hands behind your head, interlacing your fingers. Bend your knees and plant the soles of your feet on the floor about hip-width or wider apart. Relax and invite your bones, muscles, and flesh to settle and sink into the floor beneath you.

We'll start by doing a gentle side bend with the upper body. Keep your hips, legs, and feet where they are without being rigid. As you inhale, slide one elbow back toward the wall behind you and one elbow down toward your hip. Don't lift your head or elbows to do the movement, and don't force it. Instead, let your head be heavy as you slide one elbow back, creating a side bend. Then, as you exhale, slowly return to center. Aim for a soft, smooth, and flexible motion. Allow the rest of your body to shift a little if needed. Go side to side a few times, returning to center after each side bend. As you move, notice changes in your breath and the alternate lengthening and shortening of the sides of your body. Flow slowly and allow your breath to move without agenda.

As you practice, you can bring your awareness to an energetic point called Palace of Heaven (*Tian Fu*), located on the upper inner arm about three thumb widths from the armpit crease. You may feel this area gently lengthen as you slide your elbow back and move into a side bend. In TCM this point calms the Po—the part of our spirit associated with Metal—covered in the following chapter.

After five to seven repetitions, pause on one side. Enjoy a few soft breaths, feeling the expansion and gentle contraction of your lungs. Again, don't tense or push. Let your body be heavy; feel the weight of your head, arms, and shoulders release into the floor as you breathe. Next, slide your legs down and straight out; and cross the leg of whatever side you're lengthening over the opposite ankle. Inch your feet away from the lengthening side so you make a crescent moon or banana shape with your body. In this position, one side of your body will feel long, while the other will be shortened. Once you've found a comfortable position that still elicits some tugging or pressure, hold the pose for 1 to 3 minutes. As you rest in this pose, imagine your breath traveling down into your side ribs, allowing the intercostal spaces to expand outward on the inhalation. If it helps, you can place a hand on your side for a moment and softly breathe into the area you're touching.

When you have finished that side, slide back to center and then over to the other side. Cross the opposite ankle over the first, and again attend to your breath. After your second side, return to center, extend your legs, and release your arms. Notice any spaciousness or freedom in the side body, chest, or upper back.

Mindfulness of Breathing

In the Buddhist system, paying attention to the natural flow of breath (*anapanasmrti*) is taught within the first foundation of mindfulness—mindfulness of the body. In my experience, yoga practitioners sometimes find it challenging to give up trying to control their breath in favor of simple observation. During mindfulness of breathing, the breath doesn't have to show up in any specific way. We just observe with care *how* it's showing up.

As you observe your breath, it may initially seem that every breath is similar, but as you watch it, you will discover it is constantly changing along with everything else! The breath can be quiet or loud, small or big. It changes speed and rhythm, and it can affect different areas of the body. It doesn't matter what *type* of breath is appearing and disappearing. What is of concern is the quality of attention brought to the moment.

Begin by finding a comfortable position in a warm room. You can sit on a cushion or lie down with your knees bent and your feet on the floor about hip-distance apart, knees comfortably leaning toward each other. Set your timer for 10 or 20 minutes. Wear loose clothes and undo hair ties, belts, or other restrictive accessories. Begin by relaxing any areas of tension you discover. Soften your eyes, jaw, and tongue. Breathe naturally and easily, noticing the flow of breath. Allow the wind of the inhalation and exhalation to move without manipulation. Watching your breath will likely change it somehow. That's okay; just keep witnessing and feeling. Resist the urge to change it in any specific way. Breathing will happen without your control. Use this opportunity to get curious about your particular breathing style. Maintain a sense of exploration.

Now turn your awareness to your body. Feel the air coming through your nose, moving down your trachea and into your lungs. Notice how the breath affects your body. Observe your ribs moving as you breathe.

Does the breath start in one area and then move out to other areas? Do you feel it more strongly in some places? Are there places where the breath feels void or nonexistent?

Because the body's physical structures are deeply interconnected, it's possible to sense how the entire body pulses with respiration. In a relaxed, natural breath, the diaphragm knits downward on inhalation, creating a gentle rise in the belly, and then releases upward on exhalation, causing the belly to fall a little. See if you can observe this pattern in your own body. If you can't, that's okay too. Try to stay with the felt sense in your body. Rather than looking from the outside, can you feel and experience the breath from the inside? Go through 10 to 20 cycles of breath feeling the pulsatory rhythm throughout your entire body.

Next, move your attention to observe your breath's quality, pacing, and length. Without changing anything, simply notice: Are your breaths long or short? Fast or slow? Do the rate and length of your breaths vary? Or do they stay the same? Notice if there is a slight pause between your inhalation and exhalation. Do your breaths feel rough, smooth, or somewhere in between? Notice restrictions. Do some areas of your breath or body feel tight or limited in some way? Are the inhalation and exhalation the same or different? Remember to relax. Instead of chasing after the breath, allow discoveries to come to you in their own good time. Like gentle ocean waves during a golden sunset, watch the body shimmer and dance with the tempo and sensations of the breath.

When your timer goes off, give yourself time to release any concentration on your breathing and relax. You may also find it helpful to record in a journal what you've uncovered.

WORKING WITH THE BREATH

Now that we've prepared the body for breath work, we can turn to practices where we intentionally and skillfully alter the breath. If at any time during these practices you find yourself feeling overwhelmed, it's okay to stop altogether and resume natural breathing. You can also simply recalibrate your effort and engagement by backing off a bit and being a little gentler.

Viloma 1 Pranayama (Against the Grain Breath)

This practice involves controlled breath interruptions. If your breath pattern is disturbed or dysfunctional for some reason, this practice will help balance and regulate the flow of Lung Qi. In this practice, we emphasize inhalation to kick-start healthy respiratory patterns and encourage life and energy to return to the Metal element system.

We will practice three short breath retentions on a single inhalation, but remember that the number and length of retentions can vary. If it feels more appropriate to pause only once during the inhalation, do that. Or practice in a less measured way and do a breath retention a few times during the inhalation rather than at prescribed times. The important thing is that you listen to your body and breath, go slowly, and aim for relaxation. As with all the breath practices in this book, allow your pacing of this one to be natural. Emphasize receptivity and ease over strain or striving.

First, find a quiet and comfortable place to sit or lie down. Especially in cases of Lung Qi imbalance or a weakened immune system, I recommend doing this practice lying on a bolster to open the chest and lungs and aid in the free flow of breath. Start by taking deep, cleansing breaths to relax your mind and body. As we did earlier with mindfulness of breathing, use the first few minutes of this practice to notice what the breath is like without changing it.

When you're ready, inhale slowly and deeply through your nose, gently filling your lungs to about a third of their capacity. Encourage the breath to move down into the lower lungs. Pause briefly. From there, take another small inhalation, filling your lungs a bit more. Pause again for a couple of seconds. Finally, inhale again for the third and final phase, expanding your lungs to about 75 percent capacity, and pause again.

When you reach the top of your third retention, exhale slowly and completely through your nose, releasing all the air from your lungs. That completes one cycle. Start with 5 to 10 cycles and gradually increase the number as you become more comfortable with the practice. Once you have completed the cycles, return to your natural breath before slowly opening your eyes.

Cellular Skin Breathing

Find a comfortable position lying on your back with your hands on your lower abdomen or ribs. Gently relax any tension you notice. Allow your belly, chest, and shoulders to be soft. Pay attention to your breathing. Feel any shifting of your lungs, chest, and rib cage as you inhale and exhale. A big portion of the lungs comprises blood and blood vessels. As you breathe, visualize oxygen being transferred from the air to your blood through minute capillaries within the walls of the lungs.

Now sense the beating of your heart. Imagine the freshly oxygenated blood in your lungs being pumped throughout your body, nourishing every cell, or the inverse with deoxygenated blood returning through veins to the heart. Envision this flow of blood, and therefore oxygen, bathing every cell of your body through life-giving breath. Pause for a few breath cycles, feeling this flow entering and exiting your body.

Once you've connected to the natural rhythm of your breath and blood, visualize the air and energy coming into your body through your lungs *and* your skin. Feel your entire body breathing. On inhalation and exhalation, sense your whole body becoming enlivened with the breath infused with Qi or Prana. As you continue to breathe this way, begin to imagine your entire body growing a little larger with each in-breath and smaller with each out-breath. Observe which areas of the body are better at expanding and contracting with the breath.

After a few cycles, retain the breath for a few counts (or less if that is uncomfortable). After you inhale, gently hold your breath, and feel your body filling up with Qi. Continue to visualize your body growing larger every time you inhale; you may even sense the Qi growing beyond your physical body, creating a barrier around you. Slowly and gently exhale through your nose. After 5 to 10 breaths like that, return to your natural breath, relax, and notice any changes in your bodymind. Slowly conclude the practice as you roll up to a seated position.

In this chapter, we explored how our breathing and skin are intimately connected to the Metal element and some habits and practices to harmonize Metal. In the next chapter, we'll move into its subtle aspects, including emotional and spiritual imbalance and associated practices.

FIFTEEN

LETTING GO, LETTING IN

True perfection seems imperfect, yet it is perfectly itself. True fullness seems empty, yet it is fully present . . . The master allows things to happen . . . She steps out of the way and lets the Tao speak for itself. [41]

—DAO DE JING

As the crisp metallic air of autumn arrives, the horizon simply glows with grandeur. Illuminated robes of fiery red and yellow signal release as green life departs for an earthly embrace. In the flow of the Five Elements, the Metal element is a negentropic movement of dissolving and decay; it reminds us that death and letting go are just another spoke on the wheel of time. You may think loss is a harsh conclusion, but the leaves ablaze for one final goodbye tell a different story. In a reality where everything eventually declines or ends, loss is an inevitable, poignant, and even beautiful part of life. As your heart aches and your breath catches with the truth of loss, you may also have an acute awareness of the space that remains. The necessity of letting go gives you the opportunity, if you're up for it, to be at peace with a larger unknown but divine plan.

Just as the Metal organs of the Lung and Large Intestine help us physically take a breath through respiration and release waste through elimination, the emotions we associate with Metal—grief, sadness, and longing—teach us about taking in and letting go. Subtle expressions of this emotional vibration are experiences of melancholy or even nostalgia. In the body, grief causes energy to collapse or dissipate. Consider how you feel when you're sad or depressed—do your chest and heart sink inward? Grief is essentially a big sigh. When we're trapped in it, we can't take a fresh breath because we're too caved in. In Western popular culture, A. A. Milne's beloved Eeyore typifies unhealthy Metal element grief. When it's strong or overwhelming, it feels like we're suffocating or lost in a dark and downward space with no way out. A Metal element imbalance can either cause or be caused by grief that is unexpressed, protracted, extreme, or sudden.

In TCM, unhealthy grief shows up in two primary ways. Either we have trouble letting go of what has passed, or we have trouble letting in or holding on to what is of value. The Chinese characters for these two situations represent moaning and crying and a quality of hardening that can overcome us when grief is intense. The character that highlights tension has both a component for Heart and one for opposition. This suggests that when our grief is out of balance, we are denying the divine truth of our Hearts, which causes a tightening. At a high level, the Heart knows that absolutely everything has an order, but when faced with the reality of loss, our natural human tendency is to grip and hold on tight. Grief arises when we realize that we can't always hold on to what we desire, cherish, or once loved. The writer and teacher Martin Prechtel says that grief is praise of those we have lost. We grieve for what has slipped through our fingers all too fast.

Another way grief can manifest is with low self-esteem or self-worth. Rather than causing a tightening around what we don't want to lose, grief makes us tighten internally against ourselves through shame or self-criticism. In this case, we can't let in or keep hold of what we value. We may have difficulty finding the gold in life or contacting our own innate merits. Just as we need to inhale after every exhalation, both taking in and letting go keep us alive and well. Without the power of inspiration, we become disillusioned, lonely, and detached from a personal sense of spiritual alignment. Folks like this tend to experience a profound lack of meaning, isolate themselves, or give away their inner authority to something external, like a dogmatic religious leader.

Just as autumn is a time of great release, grief can also strip us down to bare bark and branches. It manifests the pain of separation from that which is of worth, and it can be a very strong state that needs a lot of time and care to heal when our loss or longing cuts deep. The spiritual gift in grief, however, is that it helps us pay attention to the preciousness of life and can lead to a profound appreciation of what we truly cherish. It also helps us recognize our *own* inherent value and supports us in giving in to something beyond or more significant than ourselves—the Chinese classics call this impartiality or righteousness. This virtue helps us recognize that there is a higher mandate beyond the ego's preferences and ideas of gain and loss. When faced with grief, our assignment as it relates to the Metal element is to eventually develop the courage to bow to our sadness, release our denial, and connect with something more transcendent. Accepting the flow of time, we "kiss the joy as it flies," as William Blake says, honoring what is cherished and eventually, after an appropriate time, finding peace and acceptance within our grief.

THE SPIRIT OF METAL

The Po, or "corporeal soul," is the aspect of awareness we link to the Metal element. Like the other types of consciousness we've discussed, this part of spirit represents certain emotional, mental, and psychospiritual qualities. The Po is unique, however, because it is a denser, earthbound manifestation of consciousness. The Chinese classics describe it as the only aspect of spirit that stays with our bodies and blends with the earth when we pass. This distinction is important because it points to how the functions we attribute to the Po are inextricably intertwined with and connected to our physicality.

We experience this consciousness when we connect to the sensate—the warmth of mindful touch, the pulse of blood, the shimmering tingle of nerve, the texture of breath. Specifically, it is a powerful symbol for the fleshy instinctual realm of our bodily tissues and impulses. Of all the different functions connected to the Po, it is primarily associated with breathing, which we worked with in the last chapter. It also governs aspects of the skin and is alert to and affected by sensation and touch. Touch is the very first sense to develop in the embryo, and in an evolutionary sense, our animal bodies are designed to crave it. As young children, we experience suckling and a caring hand as life-giving sensory input, so much so that we now know young infants suffer many health concerns if they don't receive tactile stimulation.

The Po refers to the involuntary physical responses that animate our feeling states and innate instincts, the felt sense in our bodies, and the primal intelligence living just below our conscious awareness. Someone without a strong connection to their body lives in their head or even "in the clouds." However, if the capacities we associate with the Po are strong in you, you'll have a good sense of *being* on the earth and in your body. This inner animal consciousness determines your level of embodiment. The intelligence of your Po connects you to the very core of your material nature, and since it is so closely tied to your body, it also links you to your mortality. When your hair stands on end, your skin crawls, or you have a visceral impression about a person you can't quite explain, the animal power called Po is speaking from deep within you.

Our bodily tissues are, in fact, a field of continual ongoing sensory expression. Whether feeling a slight brush of cold wind or sensing a threat, the body constantly offers subtle and sometimes not-so-subtle somatic cues that keep us safe, aware, and tuned in. For example, goosebumps, clammy hands, and blushing cheeks demonstrate momentary internal feelings directly impacting the body's surface. This blended psychosomatic reaction happens automatically. Sensory stimuli occur outside the body—primarily from the five senses of touch, taste, smell, sound, and sight—or within the body, from interoceptors signaling sensations in muscles, organs, or connective tissue. These physical messages provide critical signs of safety or threat to us and our community or tribe in response to an often uncertain and dangerous world. For instance, when a wolf pack crosses a certain threshold of proximity, a single deer will suddenly tense, signaling to the rest of the group that it is no longer safe. This sudden change in posture and affect indicates it is time to dart to safety.

Since TCM links the Po to our skin, touch, physical feeling states, and primitive or unconscious bodily responses, I imagine it governs the skin's sensory receptors. These receptors operate primarily beyond our conscious control and are connected directly to the brain through the peripheral and central nervous systems. It is incredible to realize the same primitive cells (ectoderm) that make up the brain also form the skin during embryological development. Through thousands of sensory receptors, messages of energy and impulse flow to all living tissues via nerve fibers, the spinal cord, and the brain. In expanding this idea beyond just the responses on the skin to include all sorts of sensory and bodily expressions, we begin to see the wisdom in this type of consciousness.

In Chinese medicine, the Po has a relationship with and a corresponding reflex for all primary emotions. The body speaks, whether faced with elation, aggression, fear, or sorrow. Sensations tell us when we're hungry, tired, uncomfortable, connected, happy, or irritated. The stomach churns, the breath halts, and the muscles and fascia grip when encountering psychological upheaval. Indeed, feeling states and a felt sense in the body reflect a nearly infinite range of emotions and instincts. These sensations and signals are often not immediately apparent from the outside; they are internal. Even our organs have sensory receptors that make it possible to feel and sense inside our bodies. As with grief, the problem arises when we can't balance taking in and letting go. In this case, we lose connection to space and presence in the body, and our animal sensations and responses either become numb or are concretized and frozen into somatic holding patterns rather than working their way through, which we explore in the next section.

Sometimes students don't understand how this kind of awareness that seems so material could be connected to the "spirit" layer of their beings. It's helpful to remember that many earth-based traditions and Indigenous cultures see animals as closer to nature and, therefore, closer to spirit. Once we're in a relationship with the field of presence and feeling that our Po offers us, we can relate to it skillfully and even use it as a resource. Every buzz, tingle, and pulse is another opportunity to unravel layers of ourselves formed by past habits, impressions, pressures, worries, and beliefs. The gift of this aspect of spirit is that when we develop somatic awareness of our subtle inner rhythms we gain access to greater self-regulation and unlock connection to the self-organizing and self-healing capacity we each have within.

DISTILLING VALUE

When we pay attention, it's easy to see how both taking in and letting go are natural parts of life. Therefore, if we deny either of them, we cause imbalance. The thing to remember is that they are two sides of the same coin; they work in tandem. Just like inhaling and exhaling. In a big-picture sort of way, to let in what we value and appreciate, we need space; to have space, we must let go. The inverse is also true—to truly let go, we need to have an understanding of, or connection to, something more spacious or transcendent. To connect to that sense of something greater, we need to be willing to let go. Can you see how these two are interconnected? We can't have one without the other. Especially in our modern society we don't always balance them evenly, and that's where we run into trouble.

The highest spiritual quality we associate with Metal is yi (which is different than the aspect of spirit also called Yi, connected to the Earth element we explored in chapter 12). This yi means being able to see the greater order of things, like an impartial judge. When this quality is present, you have trust in a higher plan that is beyond your knowing. In Chinese medicine, when an element is out of balance, the highest virtue or spiritual quality degrades into its linked emotion. For instance, with Metal, if I can't be at peace with a higher order, I will become myopic and grief-stricken in one of the ways we talked about earlier. In our world to-day, many people are spiritually wayward; they've lost contact with mean-ing or "something greater," whatever that might signify for them. They feel deflated and experience a lack of inspiration, hope, and reverence.

In contrast, we also live in a world that likes to hold on—to objects, people, and even life itself. On a very material level, we accumulate too many possessions, and many of us have a difficult time living minimally. Rather than focus on our own inherent worth, we seek value from ex-ternal sources. Not letting go shows up in our bodies too. Unlike animals who "shake off" their somatic responses once a stressor has passed, we humans sometimes have trouble releasing our memories, responses, and reflexes. Rather than relaxing and returning to equilibrium, somatic and psychological patterns become fixed in our bodies and start to build up. In yoga, this entrenched tension deep within the psyche and soma is a *samskara*, an ingrained impression or imprint.

Over time, not letting go causes physical, mental, energetic, and spiritual wear and tear. In my clinical practice, I often encounter patients who complain of persistent discomfort with vague signs of distress and long-lasting fatigue that don't seem to respond to conventional treatment. This tells me that the Metal element's capacity for letting go and the Po's responsibility for bodily animal instincts are out of balance. Just as we need to soften any hardening around unhealthy grief and touch into something more transcendent, we also need to disarm the somatic holding and numbing we have built up in our bodies due to our life experiences. Holistic medical systems, along with many schools of bodywork, emphasize the need to attend to these entrenched patterns deep within the soma to slow aging and maintain brilliance and vitality. We may not always follow our animal instincts, but staying in touch with them and allowing them space is key to whole body-mind health. In fact, developing somatic awareness by encouraging space and presence in the body creates a profound integration between body and mind, and it can help us tap into our bodies' innate intelligence and capacity for self-renewal. Throughout this book we explore many slow somatic practices that do just that.

We can also work with letting go by contemplating impermanence (*anicca*). Change happens to all of us, and a fundamental quality of reality is that it is inherently ungraspable. Watching your body or mind transform with aging or sickness, experiencing your children grow into fully formed adults, or losing a parent is normal and unavoidable. We live in a culture that, in many ways, denies the inevitability of aging and death. But in our effort to stay young forever, we set ourselves up for disappointment, because who can really control the effects of time? In turn, we inevitably miss out on the chance to naturally age, boldly, and with purpose. Change or loss is not always painful or unwanted, but when it is, our tendency is to resist or cling—we try to hold on rather than let go.

The Buddha's suggestion regarding the universal truth of impermanence was to observe our reactions or relationship to change closely.

He recommended that, rather than becoming attached to the circumstances of life that come and go, we accept these aspects of life as unavoidable. He said, "All conditioned things have the nature of vanishing." Time moves quickly, and absolutely everything is ephemeral, like "stars fading and vanishing at dawn, like bubbles on a fast-moving stream." Life is so precarious. Like steam rising off a warm river into the cool air at dawn, everyone and everything will eventually change. The Dharma teacher Jack Kornfield reminds us, "Suffering is like rope burn. We need to let go." When we ignore the truth of change, holding on creates another layer of suffering in the present moment. First is the pure experience of change, pain, or loss. Second is the extra "rub"—the preventable suffering that comes with denying or fighting the experience.

Really, it's remarkable we need to remind ourselves that impermanence is a part of life. The experience of change is pretty unavoidable! If you've spent any time in quiet meditation, you've surely experienced how the body shimmers with constant fluctuating waves of sensation. Wait long enough and even the most fixed feeling in the body will dissolve, move, or expand. Impermanence is also obvious in our external environment—seasonal shifts; weather patterns; the ebb and flow of politics; the evolution of civilizations and cultures; and the coming and going of work, friends, and partners. Change is the nature of life. Without it, phases of the moon would not move ocean tides, autumn would not lead to winter, and a simple seed would never transform into a majestic cedar tree. So the fact that everything is appearing and disappearing is quite ordinary.

Amid all the changes and losses, we live dazzling lives, full of infinite beauty and richness—blazing red sunsets that turn the entire lake into fiery lava, the soft skin of a newborn, a perfect lightning bolt awakening the desert sky, a secret love song sung alone by candlelight. When I studied and practiced with the yoga and meditation teacher Michael Stone, he often offered this Zen chant as a way to remember the awe-inspiring immediacy and impermanence of every moment:

Life and death are of supreme importance.
Time passes swiftly and opportunity is lost.

Let us awaken.

Awaken!

Do not squander your life.

Rather than leading to complacency or resignation, accepting imperma-nence and the fleeting nature of time can help us connect to something greater. It can soften us, help us loosen our tight grip on life, inspire us, and assist us in gaining a deep appreciation for every moment.

Embracing impermanence and learning to let go when we need to don't mean we don't deeply grieve our losses or feel pain when we lose something we desire. It also doesn't imply we shouldn't have strong goals and aspirations, which is a tricky truth for us to juggle. Of course, daily life requires engagement in the world and taking action. Humans naturally have wants and desires, and actions fueled by positive inten-tions can be full of beauty, excitement, and blessings. However, recog-nizing and accepting the natural law of impermanence and change help us release our rigid agenda for how life *should* be and aid us in experien-cing how things actually are. Feeling the grief that can accompany loss and allowing it time to heal are essential, but the key is not to become hardened. When a tree loses its leaves, it neither clings to what it once was nor anticipates what will come. Instead, the natural world is always in the flow of the ever-present now.

Think of it this way: when we investigate the nature of our bodies and minds, we discover that we hold all the elemental energies de-scribed in this book. We contain not only the dust of exploding stars in the form of minerals but also life-giving water from mountain streams, the fire of the sun, nutrition from plants, and the dirt that grew our food. Our bodies and minds are made of what we had for dinner *and* the ancient DNA of our ancestors. For better or worse, we are filled with the caring *and* critical voices of our loved ones, our education, and our past joys and traumas. Every thought arises from memory, every dream or fear is a fragment of our history, and every interaction results from the coalescence of many other innumerable moments. Instead of becoming attached to a single aspect of our experience and trying to hold on for dear life when it inevitably changes, we can be in awe of the miracle of existence itself. Ultimately, when we know everything is temporary and always changing, we are reminded of life's inherent value.

HEALING THE METAL ELEMENT

> Enjoy Savasana regularly. Set a timer for 5 to 15 minutes, lie on the floor or a yoga mat (not your bed) in a warm room, and simply let go into the limitless. Aim to release physically, emotionally, mentally, and energetically. In yoga, we practice Savasana as a way to acknowledge the immediacy and necessity of death as a part of life. You could say that all yoga seeks to attain a sort of dissolution or death—that of the fearful personal self in favor of a more universal or awakened self. It is also during times of inactivity and rest that your body-mind can let go of deeply embedded patterns, reset, and heal. During Savasana let go of your agendas and fixations and allow your body's innate intelligence to take over and seek homeostasis.

> Practice renunciation (*nekkhamma*). Rather than a rejection of something, the practice of renunciation describes a release of whatever is blocking our way to freedom and peace. For instance, in the residential retreats I offer, we often renounce using our digital devices. This helps us to simplify and quiet our minds in the service of our practice throughout the weekend. In our lives, we can also renounce things that either distract us or directly harm us and others, such as intoxicants or denigrating gossip. By eliminating these things, we have more space to breathe, so to speak. Is there something in your life that keeps you distracted or negatively affects you? What would it be like to consciously release it for a while?

> Tap into inspiration and connect with something greater. The power of the Metal element is that when we let go, we can connect to awe and inspiration because we have the space to do so. The Chinese classics emphasize how the natural world inspires reverence. Surrounded by the immensity of mountains, our conflicts and dilemmas seem small. Is there a natural place you can go that reminds you of what is supreme or beyond your self-

referential view? Consider what triggers your wonder. How can you cultivate more of it in your life?

MINDFULNESS OF BODY AND FEELING

In the following practice, we'll pay close attention to our body and our murmuring sensations. Staying present with thoughtful attention and a willingness to feel encourages us to open to all experiences sensitively and generously and to learn to live with the never-ending stream of change. We'll do this using the first two foundations of mindfulness: the body and *vedana*. The latter is usually translated as "feeling," but rather than referring to what we call emotions in the West, vedana points to the impulses or feeling "tone" within us. The word *vedana* comes from the root word *vid*, which means "to know," and is related to the word *veda*, which means "knowledge." The root word *vid* is also used in the Sanskrit word for "skin," or *vedani*, which makes perfect sense, considering the powerful sensory receptors and sensory awareness we reviewed earlier.

Somatic Movement with Antara Drishti (Internal Gaze)

As we practice movement, we can use Antara Drishti to explore and unlock habitual patterns of strain deeply embedded in the body-mind. As you move through this practice, the most important thing is to consciously practice letting go. Remember, this practice may seem simple, but it can be very profound. It's not about how far you can get. It's about tuning in to the subtle sensations within the body and alternating contracting and releasing, which is very healing and helps to reset any chronic holding. Pause after every movement and feel the weight of your body release.

Begin by lying flat on your back on a firm but soft surface, like a blanket spread over a yoga mat. Invite your body to let go. Now bring your full attention to the felt sense in your body. Feel the placement of your bones and muscles on the floor, and notice any areas that stand out to you. Don't try to discover anything special. Simply observe.

You may feel heaviness, lightness, warmth, or coolness; the movement of your breath or heartbeat; or tingles, pulses, or pressures. You may also notice fatigue, restlessness, or boredom. Allow these waves of experience to come and go. Although many qualities are arising, home in on sensation. Invite a quality of freshness into your experience, a childlike curiosity. If there are areas you don't seem to feel much, that's okay too. As you explore and develop more sensitivity, you will discover pockets of feeling. For now, simply be with what is. The task is to feel whatever is present without evaluating or categorizing.

Now turn your attention to your skull. Observe any sensations. You may notice the skin at the back of your head spreading slightly outward, accepting the support of the soft surface beneath you. There may be a feeling of air on your skin, tingling, pressure, or pain. Bring awareness to your face and neck. Once again, feel and sense. Be aware and watch every sensation without judgment. Gently rock your head from side to side, if that feels good, noticing any sensations that arise. Continue to feel your skull and neck during the movement, especially paying attention to your skull's contact with the floor.

Next, come back to stillness and transfer your awareness to your chest, back, and torso. Notice what arises. If there are distracting sounds, feelings, or thoughts, notice them, and then softly let them go, returning to the present moment in your body. You may observe the rise and fall, or expansion and contraction, of your chest and belly with the movement of your breath. As the various sensations pass through, pause, soften, and ask yourself, "What is happening right now?"

Continue to your right arm, left arm, pelvis, hips, right leg, and left leg. Notice the pressure of the floor under you and any sensations that are present. Each tickle, itch, or buzz is equal in the lens of your attention—notice them all. Finally, bring attention to your feet. Observe once again the field of sensory awareness in your feet. Listen to your body's language like a finely tuned instrument of awareness.

Next, create an X shape with your arms and legs by bringing your legs a little wider than hip distance apart and placing your arms on the floor above you in a Y shape. Place your arms at a comfortable angle that allows your forearms and wrists to be in full contact with the floor. Notice how this new configuration feels in your body.

From there, gather your attention into one foot and leg and gently push out through one heel. Keep your heel on the floor, flex your foot by drawing your toes back, spread your toes wide, and slide your heel forward. This is not a big movement, but you may feel how your foot's pushing translates into your leg as a lengthening and sliding. Feel sensations in your foot or leg as you do the movement. Perhaps you feel stronger sensations now with the engagement of muscles, which is fine, but never move directly into pain. If you feel discomfort, ease up and use less force. *Feel* the movement rather than simply *doing* the movement. Allow your breath to flow effortlessly and without manipulation. After 3 to 5 slides on one side, relax that leg entirely and try the other side.

Once you have tried both legs a few times, pause and let go of any muscular engagement. Return to a place of stillness and notice any sensation now. Perhaps you feel the echo of the movement traveling through your fascia, muscle, nerve, and bone. Simply sense and feel.

Next, try a similar movement with your arms and hands. From the X position and without lifting your arms, reach and slide one arm up and away from you as if you were doing a big morning stretch but maintain contact with the floor. Move slowly and repeat with each arm a few times: sense and feel. Perhaps there is a stronger sensation through the contact points on the floor. Don't force the movement, and again, don't hold or control your breath; instead, allow the movement and breath to express themselves easefully. Once you have finished with both arms, come back to stillness and notice. Feel how the web of skin and soft tissues reorganize as you rest in neutral. When you're ready, reach and slide the leg and arm on the same side. Repeat 3 to 5 times, then switch sides and repeat. After you've practiced both sides, pause and feel.

Now let's practice with all four limbs. Remain in the X position. When you're ready, reach and release your arms and legs simultaneously 3 to 5 times. After your final round, bring your arms back down near your sides. Soften all surface tension on your skin and feel any pulses, tingles, or buzzing from within. Remain relaxed and alert; notice the pervasive field of presence and sensation in your body for a few minutes.

If you'd like to continue with more movements, you can experiment with any other reaching and sliding that feels good. For instance, you might reach and slide opposite arms and legs, noting the diagonal pattern. After every movement, always return to a period of stillness and noticing to support somatic integration. When you're done, gently roll over and continue to remain aware of sensations as you very slowly come up to a seated position.

The Metal element is a moment of cutting back. Just as life needs growth, it also needs consolidation. We explored how this energy manifests in nature and our bodies and minds. When balanced, the qualities of Metal are pure and sharp and help us contact what is truly essential. In the Five Element cycle, Metal holds and augments Water. The transition from Metal into Water is one of deepening inwardness. In our next section we look into the season of maximum Yin—the quiet wisdom of the Water element.

WINTER
SEASON
&
WATER
ELEMENT

SIXTEEN

WINTER RETREAT & THE WATER ELEMENT

I could not bear the loneliness of being dry in a wet world. Here in the rainforest, I don't want to just be a bystander to rain, passive and protected; I want to be part of the downpour, to be soaked, along with the dark humus that squishes underfoot. I wish that I could stand like the shaggy cedar with rain seeping into my bark, that water could dissolve the barrier between us. I want to feel what the cedars feel and know what they know.[42]

—ROBIN WALL KIMMERER

Next in the ancient cycle of the elements is the mystery and hidden power of the Water element. Water is the source of all life; our bodies are made primarily of water. Life on planet earth started with microorganisms in the oceans, and every one of us began our journey in the watery realm of the womb. In Chinese medicine, Water represents our deepest reservoir of energy and greatest potential; its life-giving supply is what sustains us. The Water element in the body-mind is like an underground aquifer. It nourishes and supports you with fluids and the deepest and most stabilizing substances and structures, such as your bones and marrow. Energetically, Water also represents your innermost essence, resource, genetic memory, and power. On a psychospiritual level, when we are in touch with the highest wisdom of the Water element, we have an abiding faith in the mysterious unfolding of our lives—we trust our inborn power and the deep inner knowing held in our bones. The *Dao De Jing* highlights the qualities of Water like this:

> Nurturing the ten thousand things
> Without competing,
> Flowing into places people scorn,
> very like the Tao.[43]

As this reading implies, the masses may detest the mud and muck, but Water seeks those low places, flowing serenely through them while bringing nourishment to the earth. This characteristic is what brings Water near to the Dao.

In the rainforests of Canada's Pacific coast, a place close to my heart, Water can be seen in many shapes and forms. During the winter, a fine mist almost always clings to the cedar branches like a spiderweb. On those days, you only notice the presence of Water when you return home and realize your jacket's quite wet, even though the mist is barely perceptible. At other times, rain comes in great sheets spreading rapidly across the sky or as large droplets smacking against broad, shiny leaves. During the rainy season, creeks, streams, and ponds appear out of nowhere, feeding roots and moss with ample life-giving sustenance. What can start as a small spring somewhere deep in the mountains eventually turns into rapids, waterfalls, rivers, and streams that join with the all-important ocean. In all its states, from the icy glaciers of the high Arctic to the billowing cumulus clouds of the American Southwest, liquid, solid, or gas, Water shows us its quiet strength.

Almost every culture on earth has recognized water as sacred. Pilgrims and spiritual seekers have traveled to wells, springs, rivers, and lakes from the beginning of time for healing and insight. In Celtic traditions, springs and water wells were once seen as entry points into the otherworld—thought to be somewhere one could access a kind of magic and intuitive knowledge. Ancient wisdom traditions frequently link rivers and the water in wells to the divine feminine. In fact, in the days of early Christianity, chapels were often built on established well sites where sacred local rituals involving water took place. Following the ancient traditions of India and yoga, pilgrims gather along rivers and waterways to make offerings, cleanse themselves, and bathe. The Ganges River, the most revered of all waterways in India, is believed to be the embodiment of Ganga, the Vedic goddess of purification and forgiveness.

The dark season of the Water element is the most Yin phase of the Five Element cycle in Chinese medicine and Daoism. It is slower, inward and downward, more passive, and related to winter. It is the great exhalation, a chance to pause before beginning anew with the fresh inhalation of spring. The *Nei Jing* describes it this way: "The three months of winter, they denote securing and storing. The water is frozen and the earth breaks open . . . Let the mind enter a state as if hidden, as if you had secret intentions; as if you already had made gains . . . it is the Way of nourishing storage."[44]

The land becomes quiet and dormant during winter, animal movements slow, water turns to ice, and plants store energy in their roots. After the letting go of autumn, the winter season asks us to protect our innermost being; it's a time of quietude when we can turn inward before life picks up and blooms again. Winter, with its scent of balsam fir and cloves, is a time to move slowly, to contemplate, and to receive. This is the time of year when I long to hide out in front of the fire with a good cup of tea and a stack of books to keep me company. Perhaps at my core, I have a little bit of hibernating animal in me. Wake me in the spring to play; in the winter, I'll be in my cave, sleeping and restoring. The hush of fallen snow and long nights provide a timeless space to stop and connect with what is most important. As we allow the clamor of the outer world to recede a little, we can listen deeply and remember the light within.

Many traditions celebrate the darkest time of the year as an important moment of transition. When I worked at a rural health clinic in Nepal in late autumn, we celebrated light in a season of darkness with the festival of Tihar: homes in the village were decorated with elaborate flower mandalas, and on the third day, every entrance and window was lit with candles to welcome Lakshmi, the goddess of abundance. Pagans celebrated midwinter and the longest night of the year by burning a yule log, the ashes of which were saved for spring's first planting, a symbol of hope to come. Here in the West, many celebrate Christmas in December by stringing lights on evergreen trees, bringing the promise of new growth and renewal into the cold, dark days. In her poem "Shapechangers in Winter," Margaret Atwood describes the magical season of winter solstice like this: "The year's threshold and unlocking . . . the place of caught breath, the door of a vanished house left ajar."[45] It is a time of reflection and receptivity; tapping into this Yin energy we can sense and feel the undercurrent of our own lives. Even though winter and the Water element appear to be unproductive at first glance, all life is coalescing, regenerating, and building just below the surface. It's a time to guard and nourish new seeds of potential.

From the interiority of Water and winter, we will eventually rise rooted, ready to reach for the light, vitality, and creativity represented by spring and the Wood element. But first, we must dive into the still, dark, empty void and develop inner wisdom. Just as plants root down to rise up and break through with new growth, we also need both actions to come alive. In fact, much of the spiritual journey requires going "in and down," exploring our depths through quiet and introspective practice, not the constant "up and out" we're used to. We each must turn inward and connect to the depths where our life takes root. This inner source, our wellspring, is what gives us power, energy, trust, and wisdom. When we slow down and care for ourselves, we access this hidden well and connect with something deeper and transformative.

WATER IMAGERY AND LANGUAGE

Torrential downpours
A still, dark lake
Icicles
A clear, cold night
The new moon
Billowing clouds
Rain soaking a desert floor
A waterfall
The womb

Midnight
Shunyata (emptiness)
A deep-sea diver
An old crone
A winter festival of lights
Streams, rivers, ponds, creeks
Ocean mist
The North Star

ENERGETICS OF WATER CHART

Season	Winter
Yin organ	Kidney
Yang organ	Bladder
Tissue	Bone
Sense organs	Ears
Emotion	Fear
Direction	Inward
Sound	Groaning
Climatic influence	Cold
Taste	Salty
Color	Black

SEASONAL SELF-CARE FOR WINTER

During winter, we can heal by resting, rejuvenating, and recovering from any stressful energy outputs. It is a time to emphasize the Yin part of your nature through reflection, introspection, and receptivity. Here are a few general suggestions for balancing your lifestyle during the dark season.

> Winter is a time to restore your deepest resources. Slow down and give yourself more time to complete tasks. Ask yourself, "How am I draining my energy? Have I allowed any time to retreat from the external demands of my life, however small?"

> Relax into the impulse to rest more. Your body knows what it needs! Don't schedule too many evening engagements. Go to sleep earlier and sleep longer. Reduce or eliminate caffeine if you can.
> Slow and gentle practices are best now. However, stay active enough to keep your spine and joints mobile. Try meditation, *yoga nidra*, Yin Yoga, restorative yoga, and regular gentle walks. At the end of your practice, wear an eye mask and enjoy a longer resting pose (Savasana). Instructions for a sweet restorative pose are in Chapter 18.
> Bundle up when outside. Keep your lower back, head, chest, and feet warm.
> Treat yourself to a warm bath or steam room regularly.
> As with the Metal element's season, this is a good time to massage natural oils into your skin. In winter, pay extra attention to your ears. Read more about this practice in Chapter 14.
> Cooperate with the ancient rhythm of darkness. Turn off your house lights and hang out by firelight in the evening.
> Daytime sun exposure and spending time outside can significantly improve the winter blues. Get outside for gentle exercise every day.
> If you feel overly sluggish and need more motivation this time of year, create a schedule to keep yourself active and engaged. Book times with friends or sign up for a class.
> Use this season to feel into the deep undercurrent of your own life. What in your depths is calling you right now? Focus on that. How will you respond to the call?

WINTER KITCHEN MEDICINE

During winter, energy slows due to the influence of Cold, and the air is often light, dry, and clear. Just as trees draw their sap inward at this time of year, our energy and digestive fire concentrate in the body's core.

General tenets of winter nutrition include fortifying the whole system with hearty, warming meals containing plenty of protein and good fats. In winter, we must protect against Cold by supporting inner warmth and nourishing our Yang while guarding our fluid Yin. We do this with dense, oily foods that stabilize blood sugar and provide long-lasting energy. Winter is also a holiday season in many cultures. Therefore, place special attention on moderation and reducing any stagnation caused by heavy foods. Use these suggestions to maintain good health in the kitchen during winter:

> Eat mostly cooked foods.
> Aim to generate warmth without causing drying or overheating. Accomplish this by making slow-cooked soups, congee, stews, and broths.
> Stay adequately hydrated with warm herbal teas and hot water throughout the day.
> Enjoy healthy oils and fats like ghee, nuts, and seeds, and eat brown rice, eggs, lentils, and oats to strengthen and lubricate the body. If you eat meat, winter is the most appropriate time of year to consume animal products.
> Add sea salt and salty foods like miso and seaweed to your diet, as well as naturally sweet foods such as whole grains, dates, root vegetables, and squash.
> Cook small amounts of steamed winter greens like kale and chard, but be careful not to have too much as the bitter flavor can be cooling.
> Use small amounts of warming, pungent spices like clove, ginger, cinnamon, chilies, and black pepper. However, avoid excessively spicy foods as they dry Body Fluids and Yin, and cause excess Yang.
> Seek out dark-colored foods and foods that are black, such as black beans, kidney beans, and black sesame.
> Avoid raw and cold foods. Reduce your intake of dry foods like crackers and chips and fruit that is not in season.
> Herbal medicines at this time of year should focus on recovering from stress and deeply nourishing the body. Use tonics and adaptogenic herbs like ganoderma or reishi mushroom (*ling zhi*) and astragalus root (*huang qi*) to strengthen your body-mind and regulate the body's stress response systems. The formula Four

Gentlemen Decoction (Si Jun Zi Tang) is helpful to build Qi if you experience long-standing weakness from overwork.

As you can see, much of the energy that connects to the Water element constellates around dropping into the Yin-like depths. We can work with the Water energy present in nature and receive its gifts through seasonal food and self-care choices. However, it doesn't stop there. We can also apply our understanding to the physical and subtle body, where the Water element represents a potent center of vitality within, and to our emotions and spiritual lives, which we'll investigate in the next two chapters.

ORGANS OF THE WATER ELEMENT

As we move deeper into the body, we connect with the organs that represent the Water element: the Kidneys and the Urinary Bladder. You can find your physical kidneys by placing your hands on your lower back, just above your waist. They are situated partially behind your lower ribs. These organs filter an enormous amount of blood daily and regulate fluids. Your body can survive with just one kidney, but if both kidneys fail, you would no longer be able to eliminate wastes, and you would die.

Waste from the kidneys travels via the ureters to the bladder, a stretchable sac just behind the pubic bone that stores and eliminates urine. Together, the kidneys and bladder determine the body's overall movement of fluids and the balance of water and minerals. Some of these minerals support and create the marrow and bones. The two adrenal glands, also related to Water element energy, sit on top of the kidneys. The adrenals release hormones that help to regulate blood sugar and mineral levels, along with hormones that work together first to activate, then to counteract, the stress response.

In Chinese medicine, these two organs also maintain a balance of fluids in the body, so any issues with the physical kidney or bladder—including infections—would naturally involve the Water element. However, Chinese medicine also understands these organs on an energetic level. The energetic functions of the Bladder are similar to those of its anatomical counterpart—it transforms fluids and holds and excretes urine. The Kidneys—the Yin organ of the pair—hold extreme importance in Chinese medicine because, energetically, they are responsible for birth, growth, reproduction, and development. This means they perform many important functions to keep us healthy. Along with the adrenals that sit on top of them, they are the "root of life" or the "palace of Fire and Water"; the beginning of all other Yin and Yang in the body. Within energetic medicine, our Kidneys balance the complementary opposites of activity and rest. TCM represents this characteristic as a cooking pot over an open flame. The pot's water portrays the body's Yin and fluids; the fire below represents the Yang. The warmth of the flames steams the water (and Qi) up into the tissues and organs, where it bathes the entire cellular system and contributes to many bodily functions. If there is too much Yang in the body, the fire will burn up all our fluids, leaving behind an excess of Heat and excitation. If there is too much Yin, Cold and lethargy predominate. We need Yin-Yang balance for health, which starts with balance in this organ system.

The Kidneys are home to our potent and precious Jing, or essence— one of the Three Treasures. In its most physical form, it comprises the sperm and ovum; at its most energetic, it is our deepest life force. The potency of our Jing is revered in TCM because it determines our resilience, strengths, and weaknesses and directly impacts our longevity. We have a limited amount of Jing energy, and we maintain it with a balanced lifestyle devoid of the excesses of work, sexual output, stress, stimulants, and poor diet. Jing naturally weakens with aging, ejaculation, and childbirth. Hence, many ancient practices focused on preserving this sacred life-giving substance through sexual restraint and long periods of replenishment after giving birth. Since Jing decreases as we age, signs of aging indicate depletion—physical and mental decline, fatigue or exhaustion, premature graying, deafness, infertility, concerns with urination, low libido, weak knees, and lower back pain are some examples.

We receive our Jing from our mothers in the watery womb (similar to our genetics and epigenetics), and it combines with our fiery Shen or spirit, which we explored in Chapter 9. This joining of Yin and Yang gives us a unique template that determines our potential. In this way, the Water element represents our ancestors' accumulated knowledge, energy, experience, and the very essence and promise of who we are. However, Chinese medicine and Daoism recognize that our destiny is not entirely predetermined. To fulfill the highest expression of our unique path, we must listen carefully to the dictates of our nature and monitor our energy and activity levels. If we spend our lives overreaching or trying to become something we're not, we won't adequately preserve our Water element and Jing or use them appropriately to achieve our destiny. In that case, we risk depleting our deep essence too soon and burning out, which we explore in the next chapter.

Your energetic Kidneys govern the production and storage of minerals and blood in one of the most Yin tissues of the body—the bones. When your Water element is balanced and robust, your bones are strong; if they break, they repair quickly and easily. When your Water element is deficient or otherwise imbalanced, your bones become brittle and can easily break, often because of osteoporosis or osteopenia. A deficient Water element can also affect the bone marrow, a spongy fatty tissue within the bones that produces red and white blood cells, causing it to become soft and compromise the body's immunity. In TCM, teeth are also a manifestation of bone; frequent cavities or teeth that don't grow strong could indicate Water element weakness. The Water element and energetic Kidneys also often involve the lower back and spine. When someone comes to my clinic with chronic aches in the spine or lower back, I assess the health of the energetic Kidney and Water element along with an appropriate assessment of structural imbalance and tissue damage.

Clearly our energetic Kidneys are important! The brain (called the "sea of marrow" in Chinese medicine) also relies on a robust Water element to function optimally. We say the energetic Kidneys "fill the brain," which means that when your Kidney Qi, Water element, and Jing are strong, you will have good cognitive skills and memory. When any of them are weak, you may experience poor recall or, in severer cases, dementia. Because the Water element is closely involved in the brain's development, it also impacts cognitive maturation in children. A child who is born with deficient Jing or a weak Water element could have intellectual disabilities. I also support the Water element when working with patients who have suffered a traumatic brain injury. Interestingly, the brain does not hold the same importance in Chinese medicine as it does in Western medicine. Many of the qualities Westerners usually associate with the brain, like the mind and emotions, are instead related to the Heart and Shen (we explored this in the Fire element chapters).

The energetic Kidneys also directly influence the health of the hair and ears. Your Water element is most likely balanced if these structures and their functions work well. If you have full, healthy hair, you're more likely to have strong Kidney Qi than if your hair is thinning, dull, or prematurely gray. This is also true if you recently lost your hair due to a medical treatment like chemotherapy. Treatments like that are very depleting for the Water element and require a lot of building and nourishment afterward. If you are hard of hearing, experience tinnitus, or get frequent ear infections, take care of your Water element. We'll look at the ears and some practices to support their energetic health in Chapter 17.

Lastly, breathing difficulties (especially asthma) are sometimes related to Kidney Qi troubles. We looked at breathing in detail in Chapter 14 when we explored the Metal element.

WATER ELEMENT MERIDIANS

The Kidney Sinew channels run from the bottoms of the feet along the inner legs to the groin with branches that go internally and travel up the spine to the nape of the neck. The primary meridians also run up the front of the torso to the collarbones. The Bladder Sinew channels begin at the tops of the little toes and travel to the outside ankles, up the back of the legs and buttocks, and along either side of the spine to the crown of the head; they then descend to the face near the eyes, cheeks, and bridge of the nose, with branches to the root of the tongue, upper back, and upper chest.

To support these channels and subtler meridians associated with the energetic Kidneys and Bladder, as well as the Water element in general, we can choose specific movements and yoga postures that target the soles of the feet, back body, spine, and inner legs. When these areas are deficient or blocked, we may feel under-resourced or lacking in physical or psychological strength. When Qi and Blood flow freely through these areas, we nourish our deepest energies, relieve physical and energetic blockages, generate deep resilience for our minds and bodies, and support our overall capacity for renewal.

Sensing and Energizing the Water Element Channels and Organs

Begin by lying flat on your back on a firm but soft surface, like a blanket spread over a yoga mat. Soften your breath and let everything go. Feel the heaviness of your sacrum; allow it to release and spread. Visualize the energetic pathways of the Kidney channels starting at the bottoms of your feet and running along your inner legs. Then visualize the long Bladder channels along the backs of your legs and either side of your spine.

Take a moment and feel your bones—especially those of your lower body and pelvis. Allow their weight to sink toward the earth beneath you. Notice if there are differences from side to side. Does your pelvis feel off kilter in any way? Simply observe. Then draw your awareness to your legs. Specifically, notice the areas where the energetic channels run. Does it feel like one leg is heavier or longer than the other? Is one side more tense or lax? Take your attention up to the strong bands of tissues on either side of your spine. Once again, relax and notice. Scan each side of your body and observe. Does it feel like one side of your back is more weighed down than the other? What are the curves of your spine like? Without judgment, dive your awareness into your body and feel.

Next, bring your awareness to your physical kidney and bladder organs. When in harmony, these organs work in steady collaboration. However, with the adrenal glands sitting atop the kidneys, these organs are often overtaxed. Allow them to relax and rest. Dark blue is the color we associate with these organs of potency and Water Qi. If it helps, you can slip one hand under your lower back and place it where your physical kidneys are located and place your other hand at your pubic bone where your physical bladder lies. As you breathe, imagine a dark ocean blue permeating your Water element organs with vitality. Stay visualizing this color for 5 to 10 breaths. To exit, roll over and return to a seated position.

Next, we'll stimulate the circulation around your lower back. This is a wonderful remedy to energize Kidney Qi and stave off Cold in the body, especially during colder seasons and in colder climates.

Stand or sit in a relaxed position. Make sure your hands are warm, and gently rub the area around your physical kidneys until you start to feel warm. Once the area is warm, gently tap the area of your kidneys. Traditionally, you do this with the backs of your hands. If the area feels sensitive, skip the tapping until you feel stronger. Tap for 1 to 3 minutes. When you've finished, pause for a few minutes noting any sensations or changes.

SEVENTEEN

INNER POTENCY

We can learn to trust the relentless stripping of winter as much as the bursting buds of spring—as do the plants, taken down to bare root and then blossoming again. To agree to all the seasons and tides of awakening means that we are always walking the Way: while there are times we won't understand, there are no detours, no causes for disappointment. Though sometimes obscured by clouds, there is only the rising dawn, long and slow, that we walk within.[46]

—JOAN SUTHERLAND

The Water element vibrates with the whisper of stillness and interiority—in nature, the seasons, and the physical and subtle body. But how can we protect and preserve this important resource inside us? Now we'll explore what happens when we overtax this system leading to imbalance and some practices to regain vitality in the Water element.

WATER ELEMENT DEPLETION

Think of your energetic Water element—your Kidneys, Bladder, and adrenals—as your body's batteries. They have a strong impact on your overall vigor, libido, instinctive drives, and fears, and they're responsible for your willpower (Zhi), which we'll explore further in Chapter 18. We use and nurture our Water element energy based on our will (Zhi) and intentions (Yi), which we covered in Chapter 12. Essentially, we come into this world with a certain amount of stamina, potential, and potency—our Water element energy—but it's a limited resource. As a result, we can too easily overuse this precious energy and end up burned out. In my clinical practice, the most common way this shows up is with patients caught in survival mode—doing too much without enough rest.

You may remember that your Kidneys govern the overall balance of Yin and Yang, and Fire and Water, in the body-mind. When we misuse our willpower, push ourselves too hard, and experience too much stress (Yang)—and don't have enough rest, renewal, and recuperation time (Yin)—our Yin-Yang balance is compromised. Over time, this leads to depletion, especially of the Water element, because this element represents our deepest resources. Each of us has limited energy based on our constitution, inherited genetics, and lifestyle choices. When we drive ourselves beyond our capacity or frequently face stress, we drain the reserves that were intended to last a lifetime. Essentially, our Water element is designed to help us manage our resources and mitigate risk. On a physical and emotional level, it helps us determine whether we should step back and conserve or draw from our reserves and race to the finish line. What is vital for long-term Water element health is not to tap into everything we have too frequently.

On a physical level, our Water element is very closely connected to our stress response. When we're under stress, our sympathetic nervous system along the spine turns on, and our adrenal glands ramp up, preparing us for action. This is the feeling of being thrilled, which you've probably experienced during extreme sports or riding a roller coaster. You may remember that the Water element rules the "sea of marrow," which in part influences the health of our spinal column, fluids, and brain. In TCM, we also closely link the Water element to the emotion of fear, which we'll explore in Chapter 18. Consider how fear arises in life-threatening situations or protects us from reckless behavior. We need stress for our survival, and it can be good; the correct amount creates resilience and helps us act fast in an emergency. Ultimately, stress uses our Water element resources, but if we have adequate time to rest and replenish—and are able to return to a baseline of calm after stress—we don't usually experience any troubles.

However, habitually overusing these powerful stress hormones depletes us and pushes us to live beyond our energy reserves. When you're constantly in a state of distress, you become more prone to excess fear and anxiety, along with energy-deficit issues, sometimes called adrenal or chronic fatigue and burnout. You may feel wired even though you're deeply worn out and tired. Eventually, your body can't keep up with stress, so it adapts and lowers its overall stress response. In this case, you may notice fatigue, weight gain, slowed hormonal function, and more scenarios that indicate Water element depletion. I often see this pattern in my clinic; many people live somewhere on the stress spectrum, and their stress has ceased to be temporary.

Overwork can cause this depletion, but too much stimulating activity of any kind can also cause it. For instance, in my medical practice, I tend to see a lot of patients who are very focused on being active and physically fit. Excessive exercise or activities that demand a lot of energy output, like marathon running or frequent vigorous hot yoga, will deplete your Qi and your precious Yin reserves over the long term. I'm not saying you should never take part in these activities, especially if you enjoy them. However, if you do participate, you'll want to closely monitor your energy levels and other symptoms to ensure you're not overly depleting your Water element energy.

Let's look at another example of Water element depletion. Over the years, I've had countless patients come to me for help with symptoms of imbalance during menopause, and there are two patterns I see most often. The first involves Liver Qi, a condition covered in Chapter 5 when we examined stress that causes emotional tension and Qi stagnation. The second involves Water element energy. Frequently, imbalance during menopausal years presents as what we call empty heat signs in Chinese medicine—hot flashes, insomnia, dryness, and more. These symptoms look and feel hot, but not usually because there's too much Fire or Yang. Instead, there's insufficient Water or Yin to temper the Fire; in Chinese medicine, that's called a Yin deficiency. Without the moistening, lubricating, and cooling effects of a healthy Water element and good Kidney Qi, Fire flares upward uncontrollably, causing heat signs. If you have pushed yourself for a long time without adequate recovery and rest, you will slowly deplete your precious reserve of watery Yin energy. By the time you reach menopause, your Yin deficiency becomes more evident and the menopausal symptoms more apparent. When that happens, I encourage my patients to find ways to release stress, slow down, and nurture their Kidney Yin; I've found that the practices offered in this chapter and the next work well for them.

Remember, Water is the strength of our bones, the power of our Jing essence, and the potential we each carry inside. It is the wellspring from which the mystery of life unfolds, and without its nourishment and energy, we lose contact with what deeply supports us. When you overwork or seek too much stimulation and activity, you essentially ignore how much potency you have, lose your connection to your true Dao, and deplete your precious Water reserves. If you're habitually overextended and exhausted, get paralyzed or overreact under pressure, or experience the empty heat signs or Water element symptoms I've mentioned, your Water element and stress hormones are likely compromised.

The good news is that you can tend your Water so it's there when you need it. While you can't always avoid situations that cause stress and burnout, you can learn to protect your precious energy resources and nurture internal states of ease and presence to be more resilient when you come up against stress. Practices and remedies that support Kidney Qi can help you build inner strength. They rebuild, renew, and recover your depleted reserves and reprogram your nervous system so you can experience a lesser degree of struggle during physical, mental, or emotional challenges.

Habits to Avoid or Heal Burnout

> Know your limits. Get to know yourself and your unique energy profile. Going beyond your limits and adding too many stressors to your life make up the most common cause of Water element depletion. Don't overextend yourself or allow yourself to become exhausted by losing sleep or taking on too much. This includes physical exercise, work, and social engagements.
> Take a nap. Burnout compels us to rest and repair. Replenish the Water element through silence, stillness, and slowing down.

When depleted, it's very difficult to get in touch with your deeper knowing that will guide you to make better decisions about your energy outputs. If you tend to burn out, catch yourself before your tap runs dry. Take short afternoon naps, or practice yoga nidra daily, especially from 3 P.M. to 7 P.M. (Water element time).

> Hydrate. Dehydration is a big cause of Water element depletion and fatigue. Be sure to drink plenty of warm or room-temperature water between meals. You can also add a pinch of high-quality sea salt to your water to ensure deeper hydration and the correct balance of salts in your body.

> Nourish your body. Put a strong focus on maintaining a healthy diet of easy-to-digest foods that are warm and moist and contain adequate protein and good fat. This is essential when burnout is a concern. A diet like this will supply your body-mind with adequate energy and help you to rebuild any depletion.

> Take time for self-care. Make sure you have time every day to do something you love, even if it's just for a few minutes. Reading an uplifting book or being fully present with a favorite cup of tea can replenish the Water element. Try using natural oils on your body with the practice of abhyanga, which is covered in Chapter 14.

THE SOUND OF SILENCE

Did you know that the kidneys and inner ears develop simultaneously in utero? You might also have noticed the ears and kidneys have a similar shape. When sound surprises us, signals of danger are sent immediately from the ears through the nervous system. The ear's three fine and sensitive segments transmit sound to the brain from the outside world, but beyond that, the ancient yogis believed this sensory organ was a gateway into the inner realms and the sacred structures of the skull. In yoga, the ears are associated with the Ayurvedic element Akasha (Space) because they act as portals to the head, which is home to vata dosha. In Chinese medicine, they are the sense organ governed by the Kidneys and the Water element. Either way, the ears connect us to the boundless. They also represent our ability to listen—both externally and internally. To support these critical sense organs and touch the infinite space and power of the Water element through the ears, we need to quiet the din of distraction through intentional silence and listening.

In our noisy modern world, many of us have lost touch with the incredibly precious power of the ears. During winter and the time of the Water element, sound and silence become more apparent as the natural world calms and rests under a blanket of snow. I think many of us would agree that experiencing quiet in our loud, boisterous world is getting harder. We inundate our poor ears (and, in turn, our minds, bodies, and attention) with sounds of every type and tone on most days. This lack of silence shows up in many circumstances; it's clearly evident in our twenty-four-hour, nonstop media cycle and addiction to our devices, but it's also apparent when we can't simply listen without thinking about what to say next.

For me, quiet most often appears without effort when I'm walking in the old-growth forest near my home. Disconnected from the endless stream of noise and tremendous speed of daily life, I can drop into the emptiness and silence that hold all things. Silence helps us shift our attention away from the diversions of daily life toward the inner calling of our spirit. I believe there's a real longing for this shift; as a culture, we've lost the priceless ability to sit under the stars without a word being spoken. The Zen master Dogen said, "Enlightenment is intimacy with all things."[47] How can we settle enough to achieve this intimacy if we're distracted by so much noise? I once read of a scientific study where participants preferred electric shocks over being left alone with their thoughts! Essentially, we are a culture of thinkers and doers, not listeners. Of course, the hang glider, surfer, or hermit may touch silence more easily in everyday life, but most of the time, it seems like silence is hard to come by unless we consciously cultivate it.

Practicing intentional silence allows us to experience not only the lack of sound but something else entirely. It's interesting to note that the universe makes a sort of low-level humming sound, apparently a residue from the Big Bang.[48] In fact, silence is not a void at all. Rather, it is full, rich, and nurturing, and it holds profound potential, much like the qualities of the Water element. Thich Nhat Hanh says, "Silence is often described as the absence of sound, yet it's also a very powerful sound."[49] Like the monk, deep-sea diver, or mountaineer, we need to set up uninterrupted time to listen to this powerful sound. For instance, during the residential retreats I teach, we often have periods where we practice intentional social silence in community, which offers a unique and precious opportunity to settle the mind and cultivate an inward focus of attention. We've all had small flashes where we touch the valuable essence of silence—a moment to ourselves after a long day, a beautiful late summer sunset, some soft breaths at the end of a good yoga practice.

Sometimes, silence can even surprise us. I'll never forget the quiet awe that overtook me when I experienced the northern lights on a cold winter night in the North for the first time. Rumi describes it this way: "There is a way between voice and presence where information flows. In disciplined silence it opens. With wandering talk it closes"[50] Silence allows us to listen to something that is perhaps indescribable. It is only through quietude that we can truly stand witness to the beauty of the world and our place in it. Silence connects us to the vast mystery the yogis and sages were always pointing to, and practicing it acknowledges another intelligence beyond our small selves. When we listen to this silence, we can drop into the now and experience all that arises in the service of greater awareness and enchantment.

Listening and Bhramari Pranayama (Humming Bee Breath)

Sit comfortably and close your eyes. Arrive by relaxing and opening to what is here. Begin to breathe slowly and feel the movement as you inhale and exhale. You will notice all sorts of thoughts, moods, sounds, and sensations arising. Let them come and go. At first, it may feel like your inner world has become noisier now that you're paying attention, but in fact, you're simply noticing what's been happening all along! Whenever a sound arises, watch as it dissolves back into silence without engaging with it or creating a story about it in your mind. Gently ask yourself, "When

I strip away the narrative about what is happening, what remains?" Rest in that open, spacious awareness.

Next, gently close the tragus of each ear (the fleshy bit of skin in front of your ear canal) with your index fingers. Listen to the subtle resonant sounds of your breath as it rises and falls. To some, the sound is like a wave pulsing and flowing against a sandy shore. Concentrate on the sound and allow it to draw you deeper into yourself.

After a few cycles of natural breath, move on to Bhramari Pranayama. During this practice, you make a humming or buzzing sound to settle your busy mind, concentrate your attention, and tune the sensory organs of your ears. This practice is beneficial if your stress response has been activated and you feel slightly overwhelmed. Close the tragus of each ear again, relax the muscles of your face, and begin to hum. Make the sound even, and let the buzz from the sound envelop you. Hum for 30 seconds to a minute, or until you feel complete. When you're finished, release your hands to your legs and sit for a few minutes, absorbing the vibration. Sense the timeless current of silence that connects and underlies all things.

PRACTICES FOR BALANCE

Movements that focus on keeping the plantar fascia, lower back, sacrum, and spinal column supple, secure, and strong support the Water element. The energetic organs of the Water element—the Kidneys and Bladder—govern the balance between Fire and Water in our bodies, so using practices that balance our Yin and Yang aspects is especially helpful. Use postures such as supported and active backbends and passive and active forward bends to stoke and nourish Kidney Qi and bolster your influential storehouse of Jing. These movements also encourage greater circulation and strength in the muscles and fascia that shield the physical kidneys and adrenals. Gentle rocking movements put pressure on and strengthen these areas and pump nutrient-rich blood and fluid into the intervertebral discs to restore healthy mobility and engagement in the spine. If you experience exhaustion, choose restorative postures and avoid overexerting yourself.

THE YIN-YANG POWER OF FLEXION AND EXTENSION

In yoga, we generally consider movements that involve spinal flexion (like forward bends) Yin movements. They move us inward and are inherently more calming. Movements that take the spine into extension (like back-bends) are Yang movements; we lift against gravity when practicing them. They're more stimulating. In the practices that follow, we'll explore both types of movement to support the Water element within.

During forward bending, we stretch the thick, ropey structures of the back body where the Bladder meridians run. Energetically, the back body is your Yang protector; it acts like a shield or shell. We need the strong muscles in our back body to fire when we fight or flee. Picture how a cat rounds its back when scared—it pulls its vulnerable organs inward as a defense and uses its back as protection. Or imagine yourself running—what in your body engages? Those with athletic body types who sprint often (which is the same action as the protective "flight" response) will know the holding pattern of a tight back body well (think, restricted plantar fascia, hamstrings, low back, and erector spinae). When we're babies, the back body's strong structures help us lift our heads to see when lying prone. They contribute to good spinal curvature, and as adults, they keep us upright and ready for action. The problem occurs when tension in the back body is habitually held and rarely released, which is common when we overactivate the stress response we explored earlier.

On the flip side, backbends lengthen the front part of the body where the Kidney meridians run, strengthening weak back muscles, putting pressure on the spinal column's vertebral processes, and reestablishing healthy spinal curvature. If you spend long hours sitting in your desk chair or car, or if you experience excessive collapse and apathy, you may lose strength in your lower back and core over time. While sitting, folks frequently slump their lower backs, which causes the pelvis to move into a posterior tilt. This rounding affects healthy buoyancy in the spine and eventually causes the spine's natural curvature to degrade. If you're sitting in a chair right now, take a moment and let your pelvis move into a posterior tilt. Tip your pelvis backward so your lower back is rounded.

Observe what this does to your lower torso. Beyond influencing the health of the spine and back muscles, chronically collapsing in this way causes the compression of many vital organs in the lower abdomen and impedes energetic flow.

In either case—if you chronically overly engage your back body or habitually collapse into rounding—you may end up feeling stiff, sore, and fatigued. To remedy either of these scenarios, it's important to reestablish healthy spinal motion and movement, flow in the myofascia and meridians, and strength in the surrounding tissues. How do you do that? Begin by practicing the following movements.

Restoring Flow in the Spine

Think of this three-part undulation of the front and back of the spine as similar to a supine Cat-Cow Pose. I first learned a version of this from Tias Little; it derives from the work of Thomas Hanna and Moshe Feldenkrais. As you practice, remember that the Water element can produce so much power because it rests and goes slowly when needed. The healing potential of somatic movements like this lies in their simplicity and slowness.

To begin, lie on your back on a firm but soft surface, like a blanket spread over a yoga mat, with your arms at your sides. Bend your knees and plant the soles of your feet on the floor hip-width or wider apart. Feel your body relax and allow the weight of your tissues to drop. This is your neutral posture. Bring your attention to your pelvis and the area of your lower back. Notice how this zone feels today. Is the area around your lower back and kidneys achy or sore? Does it feel stuck or compressed in some way? Or does it feel comfortable and at ease? Simply take note without needing to change anything.

On an exhalation, press your feet down, rock your hips back, and scoop your pelvis under while gently drawing your navel toward your spine. Inhale as you slowly return to neutral. Try this a few times, returning to neutral after each movement. As you round your lower back, imagine you are lengthening the space between each lumbar vertebra.

Now, we'll try a forward pelvic tilt. Start in neutral again. This time, gently arch your lower spine as you inhale by rocking your pelvis and hips forward. Keep your sitting bones grounded as you tip your pelvis toward your tailbone. Imagine your breath traveling down into your belly; allow your abdomen to balloon out on the inhalation. Slowly return to neutral as you exhale. Do the movement a few times, returning to neutral in between.

Next, let's combine the movements into a full spinal wave. Gently rock back and forth, taking an anterior (forward) tilt as you inhale and a posterior (backward) tilt as you exhale. Aim for a fluid motion. Allow the rest of your body to shift subtly as you rock your pelvis. Move slowly and sensitively, paying attention to sensation. Observe if there are phases of the movement that feel compressed, restricted, or painful. Repeat 10 times. If you experience pain, go slower, reduce the range of the movement, and do fewer repetitions.

Next, return to neutral, interlace your fingers, and place your hands beneath your head. Begin with a posterior tilt. As you exhale, scoop your tailbone under and feel your navel pulling toward the floor. As your lower back rounds, lift your head and upper back off the floor, drawing your chin toward your chest and your elbows together, similar to a sit-up. Lower your head and body to the floor as you inhale and arch your back into an anterior tilt. At the same time, arch your cervical spine by sliding your chin upward. Practice this movement several times.

If the previous variations felt good, continue with one final version. Interlace your fingers beneath your head as you did before. As you exhale, round your spine and lift your head, but this time, make a ball with your body by lifting your feet off the floor so your knees and elbows draw toward one another. As you inhale, gently lower your head and feet, arch your back and neck, and feel your belly expand with breath as before. Practice this 5 to 6 times.

When you have finished, extend your legs and release your arms. Notice any sense of space, circulation, or energetic flow in your spine, sacrum, or lower abdomen.

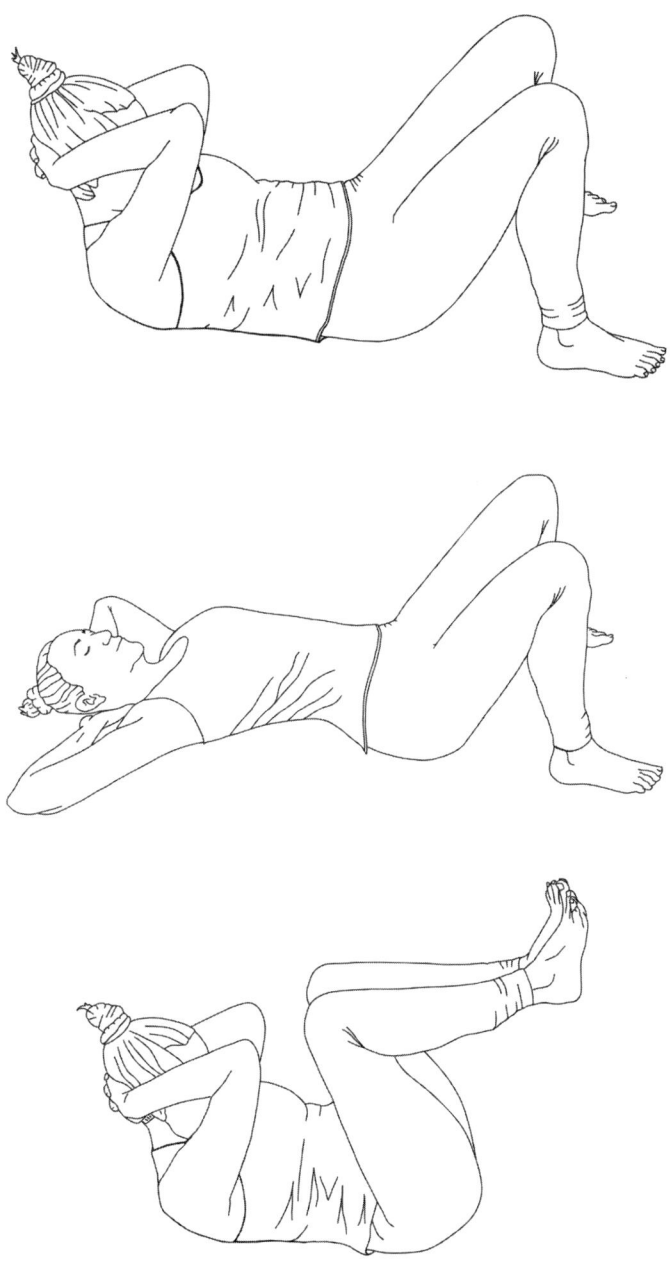

Yin Yoga Butterfly Pose

———

This is a Yin Yoga pose, which makes it a great way to practice a softer approach and build your Yin reserves. You'll want to set it up so you feel sensation, usually tugging or pressure, but nothing too extreme. Anything that feels like pain is a message to back off. Use props to ensure you're safe, but not so many that you no longer feel any pressure on the tissue. Approach your experience with mindful care, and if you feel you need to adjust or come out during a longer hold, that's completely fine; always listen to your body and modify as needed.

To practice, elevate your sitting bones by sitting on a folded blanket. Place the soles of your feet together and drop your knees out to the sides. For this variation create a wider diamond shape with your legs by pulling your feet away from your groin. Fold forward with an anterior tilt in your pelvis. Allow your spine to round (without collapsing into the diaphragm), or remain upright if you have a history of kyphosis. Rest your head on your hands, or simply let it hang, as long as it doesn't cause strain in your neck. You can also use support under your legs or knees if you have additional restrictions.

If you're avoiding folding forward or this pose causes pain, try taking the same shape lying on your back. Grab your feet in the air or place your legs and feet against a wall. This is also an appropriate variation if you experience sciatica or have any concerns about your intervertebral discs.

Once you find the variation that works for you, stay in the pose for 2 to 5 minutes, depending on your comfort level, and sense the circulation along the inner seams of your legs and either side of your spine where the Kidney and Bladder meridians lie. To release, inhale and roll up, place your hands on the outsides of your knees, and bring your legs together. Pause and notice any shift in sensation or feeling along the channels of your legs and back.

Salamba Bhujangasana (Sphinx Pose)
with Palace of Essence

Begin in the pose called Salamba Bhujangasana. Have a blanket or bolster near your yoga mat. Lying on your belly, bend your elbows so they are slightly forward of your shoulders and your forearms rest on the floor. In this position, your upper body will lift off the floor into a belly-down back-bend. Be sure your hands are out in front of you, not beside your body, and your elbows and forearms touch the floor. Maintain an equal weight distribution in your forearms and wrists. Press your arms gently into the floor to open your chest, but don't force it. Relax your neck and shoulders, and experiment with placing your legs closer together or farther apart until you find something comfortable. If your backbend feels too intense or you're experiencing any pain, shimmy your elbows and arms farther out in front of you, away from your body. You can also engage your inner thighs and outer buttocks and press your pubic bone down to create more stability and support. If you have a history of low back fragility and still feel pain, slowly come out of the posture by releasing to the floor and resting on your abdomen.

Sometimes I guide students into this pose using a fluid motion of the spine: press your forearms down, lift your chest and head on an inhalation, and feel the strong contraction of your back muscles. Stay for a few breath cycles and then slowly release downward as you exhale, sliding your elbows out to the side. Continue rhythmically lifting and releasing back down for a few cycles, sensing the elongation of your anterior (front) spine and the engagement of your back body.

After trying this several times, play with remaining in the backbend longer with support. Place your bolster or folded blanket horizontally on your mat so the long edge of the prop is facing the short end of your mat. Lie back down on your belly, resting your lower ribs on the prop. Be sure your hips are still on the ground and you feel some support from the bolster or blanket under you.

To increase the sensation in this posture, place your forearms on the bolster or folded blanket instead of the floor while keeping your hips grounded. Some students find a more dynamic variation of tucking their toes under and keeping their legs active by lifting the kneecaps and engaging the quadriceps is the best variation for them. Each option has benefits; adjust things until you feel pressure in your lower back and some length in your front body, but nothing that feels alarming.

Once you have arrived in your back-bending posture, you can bring your awareness to an energetic point called the Gate of Life (*Ming Men*) or Palace of Essence (*Jing Gong*). We locate this point near the curve of the lower back in the depression below the second lumbar vertebra. In my acupuncture practice, I use this point and others nearby to nourish the whole Water element system and to moderate heat signs, such as the ones related to menopause that I mentioned earlier. As you stay in this backbend, gently attend to the region of your lower back where this point lies by settling your awareness there in a steady but nonforceful way. If it helps, you can imagine bringing your breath to the area.

Find a place of relative stillness in this supported posture and see if you can remain here for 1 to 4 minutes—without feeling pain. (You can practice active variations for a shorter time.) Remain mindful of your breath and any sensation in your lower back as you hold the pose gently yet alertly. To release, pull the prop out and rest down on your belly. Enjoy a moment of quiet, take a few deeper breaths, and notice your lower back expanding and contracting with every breath before moving.

In this chapter, we explored how we can easily deplete our Water element and some habits and practices to harmonize Water. In the next chapter, we'll move on to its subtle aspects, including emotional and spiritual imbalance and associated practices.

EIGHTEEN

THE DEEP RIVER OF REST

When we drop fear, we can draw nearer to people, we can draw nearer to the earth, we can draw nearer to all the heavenly creatures that surround us.[51]

—BELL HOOKS

Just as winter's cold gray days cause us to become still and draw our resources close, so too does the emotion of our Water element. The emotion we associate with Water is fear. As with the emotions of each of the other elements, this one has helpful and harmful aspects. When in balance, fear keeps us safe and heightens our will for survival. Think about a moment when you had to be prepared or needed to manage your time, vitality, or money in some way. Or an occasion when you were afraid because you were in danger. Those were healthy expressions of Water element fear. As you can see, we need some fear. Otherwise, we might take unnecessary risks and harm ourselves or others. When your robust defensive instincts kick into action to protect you, that's fear's healthy vigilance keeping you safe.

Just as water can freeze, the energy of fear is cold and causes our Qi to contract. When out of balance, the general flavor of Water element fear is existential, although you can also experience it as mistrust, deeply seated suspicion, and even terror. You feel this fear deep in your bones, and when it's out of balance, you just can't shake it. To understand more about how this emotion functions, we can look at much of the language we use to describe it. We get a "cold sweat" or a "chill" when we're scared, or we become "frozen in fear." It also causes our energy to sink. In cases of extreme fear, a person may even involuntarily release urine. As with all emotions, imbalance only occurs when fear is sudden, extreme, goes on for too long, or is expressed too much or not enough. In any of those cases, it can be either the cause of Water element imbalance or an indication of it.

Trouble occurs when fear takes over our lives and becomes our dominant driving force. When this happens, either we become hyper-vigilant and overly conservative, never able to act because of fear, or we completely lack fear, which leads us to act in ways that put us in danger or exhausts our resources too early. In either case, we end up drained, isolated, resigned, or overwhelmed. One way we overuse fear is by overactivating the stress response system we learned about in the last chapter. It's also important to note that other concerns similar to fear, such as physiological and psychological issues around dissociation and numbing, can be related to fear but can also be connected to trauma or shock, often linked to Fire element imbalance (covered in the discussion of Shen in Chapter 9).

Remember, Water element energy represents our deepest potency physically, energetically, emotionally, and spiritually. It connects us to our inherited potential. When we have a healthy Water element, we use our fear wisely; we're able to stay alert and take care of our inner energy, which we then can use to fulfill our destiny. Knowing when to be strong-willed and act, even if we're fearful, and when to back off is a skill we develop as we strengthen Water. Approaching fear in this way supports the overall spiritual aim of the Water element, which is to give us access to our natural power and help us find our inner wisdom. To access these qualities, we need to slow down, rest when needed, and develop faith and trust, which we'll explore next.

THE SPIRIT OF WATER

On a psychospiritual level, the Zhi is the state of consciousness or aspect of awareness linked to the Water element. It is responsible for our most profound drives; the intuitive truth we feel deep in our bones;

our willpower, ambition, and determination; the mysterious life force that thrusts us into action. It is also what helps us conquer our fears. We maintain the health of the Zhi by delicately balancing the Yang of our instinctual drives and the Yin of restoration and repair. From a conventional medical perspective, this mirrors the functioning of the two polar ends of the nervous system—the sympathetic and the parasympathetic. We need action (Yang) and rest (Yin) to maintain well-being. When balanced, we can have a healthy relationship with our aspirations and urges while maintaining a connection to our quiet center. Mark Nepo describes it this way:

> In staying receptive, we eventually enter the paradox of everlasting will, which requires us to surrender to the unfolding of our heart, in order to discover our true strength. This lasting strength resembles a wave being brought to the surface by the depth of the sea. Each wave opens itself to the sky after being shaped and lifted by the deep.[52]

Your Zhi gives you access to the deep well of wisdom within that tells you how to use your will and resources appropriately. When you learn to stay receptive to and support your Zhi energy, you can draw it to the surface and use it to move forward with purpose and tenacity. It's like your inner sage, the acumen that helps you apply your power and resolve to self-actualize and fulfill your individual destiny. Our Zhi helps us honor and respect the energy reserves we have available and yield to the flow of our lives; it enables us to develop a healthy relationship with our highest values and stay connected to our most genuine longings without going beyond our limits.

When our Zhi is adapted and healthy, we have access to its spiritual gifts, which include this wisdom and a feeling of being well-resourced, which leads to a sense of faith in ourselves, others, and the unknown. Healthy willpower offsets unreasonable fear and gives us a sense of trust that the world is safe. We have enough wisdom to have faith in our capacities and gifts and use our resources to overcome adversities. Remember, Water is both the ending and the beginning of the great cycle. It symbolizes the empty void and the moment we are hidden away in the womb. It is unseen, Yin, and completely dark. In Chinese medicine, we develop the spiritual capacities of the Zhi—qualities like trust, faith, and wisdom—when we nurture the deep well within that provides energy, regeneration, and healing. Our current culture has rejected the watery qualities of slowness, quiet, and nondoing in many ways. Yet these qualities are what we need to replenish and support our deep reserves. You'll find practices that address this divide later in this chapter.

TRUST, FAITH, AND WISDOM

Water has enormous power and persistence, enough to carve out rock and wear down mountains. If we're not balanced, our Zhi will push through at the expense of our overall vitality. We live in a culture of fatigue. The fast-paced clip of our modern lives values dominion and results, and it rewards us for driving forward at all costs. For many of us, our lives emphasize achievement, motivated by a fearful environment that values nonstop activity. Voices are everywhere telling us to *do* more and *be* more. As a result, people no longer know how to tune in to and care for the sacred life-giving Water within; instead, they turn to stimulants, empty ambitions, and immediate gratification to propel themselves forward based on the ego's demands. Eventually, too much of this fear-driven *doing* without enough *being* leads to physical and emotional stress, a weakened body-mind, and a dried-up Water element.

Forgetting and rejecting our Yin and Water qualities parallel the rise of patriarchal structures and attitudes and the systemic oppression of the feminine. We've turned away from the part of our nature that is Yin in favor of a more Yang or masculine approach. An addiction to speed and unimpeded capital accumulation has caused us to abandon an essential aspect of ourselves and lose our subtle, intuitive ways of knowing. This has created a divide that must be healed, not only on a personal level but on a planetary level. It's not only the body-mind that suffers from the constant demands of productivity and hierarchy above all else. On a fundamental level, this daily grind causes the depletion of our vital Qi and the planet's resources. In earth-based traditions and Indigenous teachings worldwide, Earth herself is a Yin feminine being. It is this feminine mother that holds all of creation. When we deny the Yin attributes of the Water element, we also de-value the planet.

There are many ways our culture leads us away from the Water element, but there are also many ways we can return to and support this potent force. Water holds the seeds of our deepest potential, which we can only realize if we release the immense pace at which we're moving and get to know our inner world. To heal and strengthen Water, we must learn to temper our Yang ego desires with tender Yin restoration. When we connect with our internal Yin waters, we begin to favor a more sensitive and intuitive attitude, which helps us balance assertive action with nurturing self-care. In fact, tending to the Water element can be a kind of sacrifice or initiation into a new state of deeper wisdom if we let it work its magic. Only then will Water display its most important capacity—regeneration and renewal.

All living beings need periods of recuperation to sustain life. Practices that encourage slowing down and deep rest help us fill our inner well, reset our frayed nervous system, and heal our disordered relationship with fear and trust. These methods not only heal the body through tangible physical changes, but they also affect the mind. Practices that foster ease and slowing down are remarkable for stabilizing mood and encouraging a more receptive way of being in the world. Further, a slower contemplative state of mind helps us listen to and be present with the hidden, quiet, or neglected aspects of our being. David Whyte describes it this way:

> In the first state of rest is the sense of stopping, of giving up on what we have been doing or how we have been being. In the second, is the sense of slowly coming home, the physical journey into the body's un-coerced and un-bullied self, as if trying to remember the way or even the destination itself. In the third state is a sense of healing and self-forgiveness and of arrival. In the fourth state, deep in the primal exchange of the breath, is

the give and the take, the blessing and the being blessed and the ability to delight in both. The fifth stage is a sense of absolute readiness and presence, a delight in and an anticipation of the world and all its forms; a sense of being the meeting itself between inner and outer, and that receiving and responding occur in one spontaneous movement.[53]

As previously discussed, healing the Water element involves learning to trust in the natural unfolding of our lives and not "push the river." From the Daoist perspective, this is called *wu wei*, or effortless action. Essentially, when the Water element is vital and robust, we realize the wisdom that involves less *doing* and more *being*. Lao Tzu says in the *Dao De Jing*, "Nothing in the world is as soft and yielding as water. Yet, for dissolving the hard and inflexible, nothing can surpass it. The soft overcomes the hard; the gentle overcomes the rigid."[54] When we cultivate the Water element, we tap into a force far greater than our fiery drive or our fearful nature. We draw on the profound mystery at the center of who we are.

It's a radical act these days to pause and practice wu wei. Practices that encourage us to stop the constant forward-driving momentum fly in the face of our results-focused world, but they are exactly what we need. Developing healthy willpower can help you find the middle way between striving toward your goal regardless of the consequences and leaving everything up to fate. It can help you contact the source or Dao itself, being able to flow *with* life instead of against it. In this way, your Yin reserves support greater resilience, help you to trust your path, and are always there to support you in the long term like a wellspring.

As long as we're physically and mentally safe, healing the psychological and spiritual aspects of the Water element requires getting comfortable with the unknowable parts of life. We awaken to the unpredictability of life every day, not knowing how things will turn out. Instead of immediately leaping into action or collapsing in despair, can we allow ourselves to not know? Too much certainty can lead to narrow-mindedness, complacency, and a lack of open curiosity that hampers spiritual progress. However, being okay with some fear and having faith in not knowing help us access the openness that is usually beyond the conditioned mind. The wisdom of the Water element tells us it's okay to trust in the unknown; intuition, creativity, and potency are available there. Ultimately, the Water element asks us to relax into the mysteries of life and be open to awe, to have faith and trust in something deeper than our personal motives and agendas. It's fine, of course, to not know or have every answer. At those times, the watery well of your being can sustain you through winter hibernation, and soon enough, spring will return.

In fact, not knowing can be a powerful gift. A well-known story in the Zen tradition highlights this concept. One day, a Zen monk named Dizang sees his friend getting ready to leave on pilgrimage and asks him, "What is the purpose of your pilgrimage?" His friend replies that he doesn't know, to which the Zen monk nods and responds, "Not knowing is most intimate." Many fears, preconceived ideas, plans, and projects typically burden us, yet so much about our experience is unknown. When we embrace this truth, we can relax a bit and slow down. We get closer to this very moment and realize all experience is uncertain. Facing the death of what you know requires trust in your resources. This trust is not blind; it depends on a settled nervous system and wisdom cultivated through slowing down, which we explore in the practice section of this chapter.

This body-mind, and all of life, is an ever-flowing river. Like mist evaporating on a mountain peak or a quickly melting ice-cream cone, all things are inherently ungraspable. Instead of floating adrift in this ever-fluctuating tide or becoming dried up by all the stress and activity of change, we can learn to anchor to a timeless internal resource through meditation and rest. These practices teach us to settle the buzz and drop below the surface waves into a place of infinite depth, silence, and stillness. In yoga and the meditative arts, the ultimate expression of this is *samadhi*, usually translated as "meditative absorption." The Buddha says, "A mind that has *samadhi*, a mind that is gathered, will naturally see things the way they actually are and be freed from confusion."[55] When you have a collected mind, you can access your vast inner resources and follow your deeper flow instead of being swept up in the next swift-moving current. Practices like restorative yoga and meditation can train your mind to ride the waves of sensation, thought, and emotion with trust. You learn to notice what is happening and be with whatever is unfolding to fully experience all things. From this place of presence, your true wisdom shines through the darkness.

HEALING THE WATER ELEMENT

> Practice nondoing. Rather than forcing things to happen, can you drop into the natural flow of things? Effortless effort, or wu wei, can help us develop the positive or spiritual qualities of Water. Think about all the activities and roles you're engaged in. What would it be like to suspend the need to do and fix, and instead just be with what is as it is? Aim to observe when you're not in this flow state and when you are. Ask yourself, "How do those times feel? Is there a state of body, mind, or heart that is especially present?" Remember that much of your body is made of water. Consider how you can embody flow more often in your life and in your yoga and meditation practice. Use the relaxation practice in the practice section to investigate wu wei further.

> Slow down and develop concentration. In yoga, the Sanskrit word used for concentration is *dharana*, which comes from the root *dhr*, meaning to "hold" or "support." Whether it's for five minutes at your desk in the middle of a busy day or a longer formal meditation, expand your capacity for stillness by holding your attention on a single object of attention like your breath. Refer to the samatha practice in this chapter or the mindfulness instruction in Chapter 14 for more information.

> Get to know your fear. As the emotion most closely linked to the Water element, fear can stop us in our tracks and protect us when needed. Consider how fear manifests in your life. Do you experience fear as a huge wave that overtakes you or a slowly rising flood? Does urgency related to fear motivate your choices regarding finances, relationships, or work? Contemplate how you might be losing energy because of your fear and, conversely,

how fear might be protecting you. Are there ways you would like to let go of fear? Or maybe ways you can build more vigilance to safeguard your resources?

> Spend time in quiet reflection contacting your inner wisdom. Notice what happens when your Water element is out of balance and you use your Zhi too much or not enough. What happens when you let your ambitions take over? What happens when you don't have any drive? Do you become depleted and dried up like a desert without rain? Or stagnant and murky like a dark, damp swamp? Offer yourself presence and see what emerges. To heal the Water element we pause with trust, not fear. Once you are feeling present with yourself, ask your still quiet center, "Am I using the resources available to me appropriately? What remains beyond my roles and responsibilities? What is absolutely essential? What is really true for me beyond the doing and busyness?"

Restorative Savasana

———

I once heard Judith Lasater (one of the creators of modern restorative yoga) say, "Speed is the enemy of relaxation." How true that is! Take your time with this posture—it involves *a lot* of props (and they're not optional), but it's worth it. Slowing down to tend to your body-mind is central when working with the Water element. Be sure to place the props just right so you don't experience any agitation in the pose. The name of the game here is deep-supported relaxation. This pose should not be challenging or cause a "stretch"; instead, aim for comfort and gentle opening. Be sure you're warm and in a quiet, distraction-free environment for this delicious gift to yourself. I find this posture especially helpful for fatigue and exhaustion; it's also great to "top up" your watery Yin reserves daily or whenever you need a boost. Plus, it can help reset your nervous system and counteract your stress and fear response.

Start by placing a bolster lengthwise on your mat. Prop up one end of the bolster so it is at a 45-degree angle to the floor. This angle will ensure the parasympathetic response is adequately triggered. You can use blocks, another bolster, couch cushions, or rolled blankets to accomplish this. Place another bolster (or a rolled blanket) horizontally on your mat under your knees, and roll a smaller blanket under your Achilles tendons. Place two more props on either side of the original bolster to elevate your arms; blankets or cushions work well for this. Be sure to have a spare blanket behind your head and one to cover yourself. Finally, you'll need a small eye pillow or face cloth to cover your eyes.

Sit in front of the lower end of the main bolster and lie back so your knees and Achilles tendons rest comfortably on their supports. Arrange the blanket under your head and upper back so your upper back is supported and your forehead is slightly higher than your chin. Tuck the blanket around both sides of your head, creating a cradle for your skull. Rest your arms on their props so your wrists are higher than your elbows, and your hands can relax on your abdomen. Set a timer for at least 10 minutes. Finally, drape a blanket over yourself and cover your eyes. Just as water obeys gravity, sink and surrender your weight into the support and comfort of the props. Make minor adjustments until there is no nagging discomfort. Relax any tension in your belly, jaw, or shoulders, and soften your breathing. Observe sensations arising and dissolving as if they were ripples on the surface of a pond.

Most importantly, let go. Rest knowing there is nothing to do but relax. When your timer goes off, move slowly to transition. Roll to one side, and use your arms to gradually push yourself up, with your head coming up last. Sit for a moment and feel the space and peace you've created.

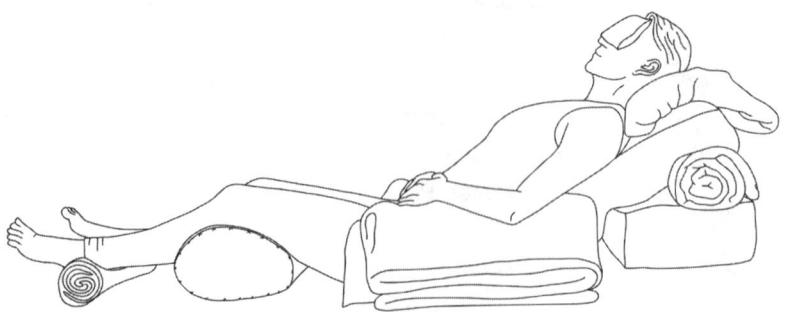

Samatha Meditation

Samatha, usually called calm abiding, is a foundational meditation method that helps quiet the body-mind and intensify presence through steady but gentle concentration. Use this practice daily to settle stimulation and distraction or whenever you need to reset and touch the depth of support the Water element provides.

Begin by finding a comfortable seat. Set your timer for 10 or 15 minutes. Keep your spine tall and place your hands palms-down on your legs. Close your eyes or simply soften your gaze. Soften your belly and relax your shoulders, eyes, jaw, and tongue. As you settle, take a few deeper breaths. Invite your lower body to descend. After a few moments, gather your attention on your breath. During samatha practice, we clarify and strengthen awareness by gently concentrating on a single point and intentionally sustaining a focus. As you sit, watch the movement of your breath. Feel yourself inhale and exhale with a light but steady attitude. Observe how the breath comes and goes: here one moment, gone the next. Remain anchored on your breath as thoughts and feelings rise and fall. When you observe your mind wandering away from your breathing, gently return your attention without judgment. Note the next wave of breath. Some breaths may be deep, others shallow. Some long, others short. It's not about changing your experience in any way. Simply watch this steady coming and going. When the timer goes off, slowly open your eyes and return.

Inner Trust Meditation

To begin, find a comfortable position, sitting upright or lying down—whichever feels better. Close or soften your eyes; relax and enjoy a few full breaths. Invite your mind and body to arrive here. Recognize this transition between your outer life and your internal practice. Imagine now that you're settling attention deep inside your bones. Feel heaviness in your hips, thigh bones, and feet. As you collect your attention on these

Yin Water element structures, let go of thinking about and striving toward the future.

From here, draw your attention down to your lower abdomen. Relax any tensing or gripping that you notice. Soften your breath and observe the slight rise and fall of your lower belly as you breathe. Spend a few minutes here, relaxing and breathing. Then take your attention to your kidneys at the lower to midback on either side of your spinal column. Imagine you're breathing into all the structures of your lower back. Watch any movement occurring from the rise and fall of your breath, concentrating your attention in and around the physical organs of your kidneys. Sense the energy held within these storehouses of Qi and deep vitality. This is where much of your Water element power lies. Once again, take a moment to be here now—acknowledge there are situations, realities, and circumstances that are currently unknowable. Reflect on a situation in your life where you don't have all the answers right now. Or perhaps consider the more significant truths of life, like old age, sickness, and death. Feel the poignancy of the unknown—we simply cannot always know everything. Return your attention to the centers of your lower belly and lower back. Feel your breath and notice what it's like not to know while remaining connected to these centers. Can you settle into the not knowing?

Now turn toward the opposite, the concrete. How does it feel in your belly, back, and bones? How does it feel to trust that this is your body, this is your breath? How does it feel to know you are here now? Allow this quality of presence to sink deep inside. Feel the steadiness and support of your belly center and lower back as you watch your breath flow. Ask yourself what else you know and can trust while remaining open to not knowing. Imagine your reflection has appeared in a pool of water in front of you. Ask yourself what is genuinely worth the precious and easily depleted resource of energy inside? What is whispering to you below the surface of your life? Your most profound wisdom comes from trust and inner listening. Honor what is true for you now. Stay quiet a while longer, remaining receptive to any other messages arising from the deep. When you're finished, spend a few minutes journaling about any insight that came to you.

The Water element expresses a time of maximum Yin. In the wheel of change, its qualities flow downward and inward. We've explored how Water's wisdom is manifest in nature and our bodies and minds. When balanced, it is powerful and fluid. In the Five Element cycle, Water feeds the new growth of Wood, and so the cycle continues. With each repetition of the cycle, the seasons remind us of the importance of every phase. Learning to pivot direction when needed, and honoring times of moving inward or outward, may we remember to listen to these influential cycles of the earth and rely on them to guide our way.

EPILOGUE

*I came to realize that mind is no other than mountains and rivers
and the great wide earth, the sun and the moon and the stars.*
—DOGEN ZENJI

What does it mean to follow the wisdom of the body and earth? We've explored how the ancient healing arts of yoga, Ayurveda, Daoism, and Traditional Chinese Medicine help us reveal, relate to, and heal both familiar edges of experience and undiscovered depths. Working with these wisdom traditions not only has clear physical, energetic, mental, and spiritual benefits but also helps us develop a more inclusive, expansive, and illuminated view of ourselves and our place in the world.

By now you may have felt or experienced how becoming aware of seasonal rhythms is a powerful way into this perspective. These wisdom traditions highlight how our elemental kinship with the natural world can guide us into a more fruitful relationship with ourselves and a deeper understanding of the many patterns affecting all things. Natural laws connect you to the breathing trees, flaming sun, rich soil, mountain peaks, and sparkling creeks. Whether it's spring, summer, autumn, winter, or the interchange between seasons, your body, mind, and spirit reflect the play of warmth and shadow, sky and sand, stars and sun. We are each an integral part of the living, breathing body of the earth. When we align with natural rhythms using body-centered awareness, the optimal conditions for physical health, contentment, and joyful living arise naturally.

We also explored new horizons in our inner expanse. Our physical and subtle bodies support our activity and keep our energy levels stable yet flexible; our minds and emotions direct our feelings, thoughts, and intentions; and the spirit of our Heart guides and lights our way. When we attend to all these essential parts, we bolster our unique strengths and gifts for our journey through life. Our path, or Dao, is nourished and upheld by these various realms of our being if we know to care for them skillfully. Once we learn to consciously relate to ourselves in this way, making choices that promote health becomes easier and more natural. Rather than a strict set of rules, nourishing life (yang sheng) becomes a habit of increasing subtlety that we can tweak depending on what is currently needed.

Likewise, once we see ourselves as the multifaceted beings that we are—including physical, subtle, mental, emotional, and spiritual aspects—we more readily perceive how these complex bodies and minds that once felt so separate are profoundly connected to a much vaster whole. The traditions we've been exploring tell us that as we walk our unique Dao, our task is to recall our deep interconnection, internally and externally, and therefore remember our true nature.

In Daoism, the ancient method of energetic cultivation, *Nei Dan* is translated as "inner work" or "alchemy." However, rather than turning base metals into gold, it is a practice in which internal refinement leads to eventual transformation or self-realization. This development supports the capacity for an awareness that is not divided or fractured. In Sanskrit, we use the word *advaita*, meaning "without division" or "nondual." This undivided state of wholeness and inner wakefulness never goes away. It is our stablest ground; we can always return to it.

You may remember that Dao itself is not only a path or route; it also refers to the all-encompassing empty unknown. We've learned how this emptiness is not vacant. The paradox is that it is incredibly full. Just like Yin and Yang exist in relationship—transforming, sustaining, and harmonizing one another—emptiness and fullness preserve and maintain each other. As we become more integrated, undivided, or cohesive, we naturally experience this original nature and our inherent interdependence with all things.

While writing this book, I often walked and sat in the woods in between writing periods. Lying on my back and staring up at the outline of branches in the silver sky above me, I would contemplate: What is it that this wild earth wants to tell us? And how can we make a difference when faced with the immensity of our problems? In a time when many people feel spiritually adrift and alone in a world of endless sound bites vying for attention, we must remember our sacred belonging: connection to ourselves and the bond we have with the whole living world. No matter how much the dominant culture encourages a forgetting of this fundamental connection and tries to replace it with a kind of egotistic hyperindividualism, the fact remains that we can't go it alone. In nature, nothing thrives on its own. The rivers, rocks, forests, plants, and animals all operate within a mutual support system to ensure collective survival.

If you're interested in seeking out the holistic healing arts, your path of study and practice may, for a long while, focus on developing good health and shoring up a robust sense of self, especially if you are facing health challenges or experiencing low self-worth, as many people in the West do. However, eventually, it is imperative that our practice not only serve us but also be for the benefit of all. Realizing this, we can move beyond our painful isolation and instead cultivate conscious awareness of a relational field. As we recall our relationship to the larger fabric of life, we might slow down and make better choices. We can recognize the importance of every small act and become a clearer force for good in the wider world. Living in a culture obsessed with grand gestures and sensational stories, I feel there is something magical and radical about emphasizing the importance of small daily choices. Joanna Macy reminds us, "When you act on behalf of something greater than yourself, you begin to feel it acting through you with a power that is greater than your own."[56]

It is a buoy to know that the traditions we've been investigating were not generally developed in times of simple peace and prosperity. In many cases, the teachings and practices we've explored were codified during periods of extreme upheaval and social stratification. Perhaps, then, we're not so alone in dealing with our many troubles. We have the guidance of the ancients who have walked the path before us and created detailed instructions to follow. When the problems of our beautiful world seem insurmountable, this clarifies my way and gives me courage for the road ahead.

When I teach Chinese medicine, I often remind students that we learn the principles of TCM best when we approach them in a circular fashion rather than a linear one. Just as each season relies on the one before and after, remember that each principle we've touched on is made richer the more the whole picture comes into view. Even after many years of immersion into these topics, every time I revisit a familiar concept, new layers of meaning are revealed. The map of the ancients is not linear, but it is not entirely circular either. Instead, this route is a spiral path with branches reaching up and down. In Daoist terms, this guide helps us stand between heaven and earth. We may return to specific seasons or life lessons again and again, but with every iteration, we are different. Engaging with these ideas and practices is a lifelong voyage of deepening discovery.

As we come to the end of our journey, we might remember that a moment of pause is another fundamental rhythm in nature. As we continue to walk our path and meet the many challenges, joys, and sorrows of our time, I encourage you to pause and remember that effective action comes from staying connected to your still empty center—your Dao, which is ultimately guided by the light of your Heart. Being more connected is not about ignoring your pain or the world's difficulties. Rather, it's about learning to dance with them and live with authenticity. It's been an absolute joy to share just a small piece of these sacred traditions with you. If you would like to learn more, I invite you to join me at jenniferraye.com and wisdomofthebodybook.com for more information and resources. I hope you return to these concepts for many years to come and that the gifts they offer continue to support you on your path.

May you be well in body, heart, and mind.
May you be at peace internally and externally.
May you be healthy, vital, and free.
And may you *always* know your true nature.

ACKNOWLEDGMENTS

Many sources of support nourished me during the creation of this book. First, I would like to thank my family—my parents who always encouraged me to follow my path and my sister who has always been by my side. Also, my dearest friend, dedicated husband, and life partner, Kristofer. I wouldn't be the writer, teacher, or woman I am today without his unwavering support and love. Extra gratitude to Kristofer for contributing the book's helpful illustrations.

A very special thanks to the whole team at Shambhala Publications—especially my editor, Beth Frankl, for her patient, clear, and kind guidance, and for believing in and championing this project from the beginning. Thank you for making this dream come true. Additional thanks to Samantha Ripley and Karen Steib, and all others involved in the publishing process including Daniel Urban-Brown for the beautiful cover design. Many thanks to Linda Sparrowe for guiding me in so many facets—her enthusiastic encouragement, keen eye, and inspired suggestions and edits made this book possible and made me a better writer in the process. Thank you.

This book is the summation of decades of study and practice with countless teachers, mentors, and healers, many of whom I was lucky to meet at a young age. Most notably, I would like to thank Tias and Surya Little—their dedication, care, and encouragement have had a significant impact on my practice and teaching. Special thanks to Tias for his very generous contribution in writing the foreword for this book. I would also like to thank my Buddhist teachers, especially Thanissara and Kittisaro, whose grounded presence and openness helped me come into a steadier relationship with myself. Additional thanks to Jill Satterfield, whose kind encouragement helped me find my voice. Also, gratitude to Spirit Rock Meditation Center and the many other movement, meditation, and bodywork instructors too numerous to name who touched my life and guided and influenced my work.

Appreciation to my academic teachers, including my women's studies professors who helped me see the world more clearly and develop my writing. Thanks to my early herbal medicine and healing foods teachers who sparked a passion in me, including Dr. Terry Willard and Paul Pitchford, as well as my Ayurvedic and Chinese medicine teachers, especially Dr. Kevin Hu and Dr. Reuven Freesman. I would also like to thank my friend and mentor Andrew Schlabach, who inspired me to look deeper while practicing in Nepal. A special thanks to Todd Howard for always having an open door and offering me a teaching position all those years ago. I have had the good fortune to study with and be influenced by many other wise practitioners and teachers whom I'd like to thank for their scholarship, including Lorie Eve Dechar, Lonny Jarrett, Vasant Lad, Dr. Claudia Welch, Elisabeth Rochat de la Vallée, and Jeffrey Yuen.

Profound gratitude to all those who have supported my work over the years and those who work in my business from behind the scenes. Heartfelt gratitude to the many yoga studios and retreat centers around the world who have hosted me, especially those at the lovely Stowel Lake Farm. To my wonderful patients, students, and readers—thank you for showing up with your endless curiosity and insights. Your presence in my life is a true gift.

Writing this book has also renewed my sense of awe and appreciation for the traditions themselves—the endless wisdom of the Buddhadharma and all those physicians, sages, and yogis who walked this path before me. I am eternally indebted and have immense gratitude for these wisdom keepers. Lastly, my biggest inspiration of all: the land. To the animals, the trees, mountains, and streams—thank you.

NOTES

1. Lao Tzu, *Tao Te Ching*, trans. John C. H. Wu (Shambhala, 2006), 121.
2. Lao Tzu, *Tao Te Ching: An Illustrated Journey*, trans. Stephen Mitchell (Frances Lincoln Ltd., 2013), verse 1.
3. Lao Tzu, *Tao Te Ching: An Illustrated Journey*, verse 23.
4. Paul U. Unschuld, Hermann Tessenow, and Zheng Jinsheng, *Huang Di Nei Jing Su Wen: An Annotated Translation of Huang Di's Inner Classic—Basic Questions* (University of California Press, 2011), 1:443.
5. Lao Tzu, *Tao Te Ching: A New Translation*, trans. Sam Hamill (Shambhala, 2007), 4.
6. Paul U. Unschuld, *Huang Di Nei Jing Ling Shu: The Ancient Classic on Needle Therapy* (University of California Press, 2016), 257.
7. Jeffrey Yuen, "Dao Yin Sinew Releases," Daoist Traditions College, October 28, 2022.
8. Unschuld et al., *Huang Di Nei Jing Su Wen*, 1:56.
9. Unschuld et al., *Huang Di Nei Jing Su Wen*, 111.
10. Lao Tzu, *Tao Teh Ching*, trans. John C. H. Wu (Shambhala, 2006), 65.
11. "Etymology of Emotion," Online Etymology Dictionary, updated February 18, 2025, https://www.etymonline.com/word/emotion.
12. John Knoblock and Jeffrey Riegel, trans., *The Annals of Lü Buwei* (Stanford University Press, 2001), 66.
13. David Whyte, *The Bell and the Blackbird* (Many Rivers Press, 2018).
14. Judith Berger, *Herbal Rituals* (St. Martins, 1998), 67.
15. Unschuld et al., *Huang Di Nei Jing Su Wen*, 1:45.
16. Mary Oliver, *Upstream* (Penguin Press, 2016), 7.
17. Swami Muktibodhananda, *Hatha Yoga Pradipika* (Yoga Publications Trust, 1993), 208–12.
18. Lao Tzu, *Tao Te Ching: A New Translation*, 111.
19. This quote is used by many activist organizations and was popularized by the Zapatista movement in the midnineties. It was originally written by Greek poet Dinos Christianopoulos in 1978. It was translated into English by Professor

Nicholas Kostis (1995) in a collection titled *The Body and the Wormwood* (1960–1993).

20. Sarvepalli Radhakrishnan, *Principal Upanishads* (George Allen & Unwin, 1968), 203.

21. Richard Wagamese, *Embers: One Ojibway's Meditations* (Douglas & McIntyre, 2013), 46.

22. Unschuld et al., *Huang Di Nei Jing Su Wen*, 1:46.

23. Unschuld et al., *Huang Di Nei Jing Su Wen*, 155.

24. Krista Tippett, host, *On Being with Krista Tippett*, podcast, "John O'Donohue: The Inner Landscape of Beauty," The On Being Project, original broadcast February 28, 2008, last updated February 10, 2022, https://onbeing.org/programs/john-odonohue-the-inner-landscape-of-beauty.

25. Unschuld, *Huang Di Nei Jing Ling Shu*, 756.

26. Elizabeth A. Johnson, *Women, Earth, And Creator Spirit* (Saint Mary's College, 1993), 39.

27. Giovanni Maciocia, *The Foundations of Chinese Medicine: A Comprehensive Text for Acupuncturists and Herbalists* (Elsevier Churchill Livingstone, 2005), 69.

28. Jack Kornfield and Paul Breiter, *A Still Forest Pool: The Insight Meditation of Achaan Chah* (Quest Books, 2012), vi.

29. John Blofeld, *The Zen Teaching of Huang Po: On the Transmission of Mind* (Grove Press, 1984) 93.

30. Pema Chödrön, *Comfortable with Uncertainty: 108 Teachings on Cultivating Fearlessness and Compassion* (Shambhala, 2003), 1–2.

31. Robin Wall Kimmerer, *Braiding Sweetgrass* (Milkweed Editions, 2013), 337.

32. Sharon Salzberg, "How to Foster Equanimity: Sit Like a Mountain." *Lion's Roar*, last modified August 28, 2015, https://www.lionsroar.com/how-to-foster-equanimity.

33. Alper Evrensel and Mehmet Emin Ceylan, "The Gut-Brain Axis: The Missing Link in Depression," *Clinical Psychopharmacology and Neuroscience* 13, no. 3 (2015): 239–44.

34. Léon Wieger, *Chinese Characters: Their Origin, Etymology, History, Classification and Signification: A Thorough Study from Chinese Documents* (Paragon Book Reprint Corporation, 1965), 187.

35. Unschuld, *Huang Di Nei Jing Ling Shu*, 148.

36. Thanissaro Bhikkhu, trans., "Yamakavagga: Pairs" (Dhp I), Access to Insight (BCBS Edition), November 30, 2013, http://www.accesstoinsight.org/tipitaka/kn/dhp/dhp.01.than.html.

37. Arundhati Roy, *An Ordinary Person's Guide to Empire* (Penguin Books, 2005), 44.

38. Unschuld et al., *Huang Di Nei Jing Su Wen*, 1:47–49.

39. Pema Chödrön, *When Things Fall Apart: Heart Advice for Difficult Times* (Shambhala, 2000), 7.

40. Sam Hamill and J. P. Seaton, trans., *The Essential Chuang Tzu* (Shambhala, 1999), 42.

41. Lao Tzu, *Tao Te Ching: An Illustrated Journey*, verse 45.

42. Kimmerer, *Braiding Sweetgrass*, 295.

43. Lao Tzu, *Tao Te Ching: A New Translation*, 11.

44. Unschuld et al., *Huang Di Nei Jing Su Wen*, 1:49–50.

45. Margaret Atwood, *Morning in the Burned House* (McClelland & Stewart, 1995), 124.

46. Joan Sutherland, Roshi, "Embracing Change: Seasons of Awakening," https://www.eomega.org/article/embracing-change-seasons-of-awakening.

47. Jakusho Kwong, *No Beginning, No End: The Intimate Heart of Zen* (Shambhala, 2010), 153.

48. Richard Rosen, *Pranayama beyond the Fundamentals* (Shambhala, 2006), 118.

49. Thich Nhat Hanh, *Silence: The Power of Quiet in a World Full of Noise* (HarperCollins, 2015), 8.

50. *The Essential Rumi*, trans. Coleman Barks (Castle Books, 1997), 32.

51. bell hooks, "bell hooks and John Perry Barlow Talk 'Prana in Cyberspace,'" *Lion's Roar*, September 9, 2022, https://www.lionsroar.com/bell-hooks-talks-to-john-perry-barlow.

52. Mark Nepo, *Drinking from the River of Light: The Life of Expression* (Sounds True, 2019), 34.

53. David Whyte, *Consolations: The Solace, Nourishment and Underlying Meaning of Everyday Words* (Many Rivers Press, 2014), 182–83.

54. Lao Tzu, *Tao Te Ching: An Illustrated Journey*, verse 78.

55. Kittisaro and Thanissara, *Listening to the Heart: A Contemplative Journey to Engaged Buddhism* (North Atlantic Books, 2014), 49.

56. Joanna Macy, "The Great Turning: An Interview with Joanna Macy," *Yes Magazine*, April 1, 2000, https://www.yesmagazine.org/issue/issues-new-stories/2000/04/01/the-great-turning.

REFERENCES

Agnivesa. *Charaka Samhita*. Translated by Ram Karan Sharma and Vaidya Bhagwan Dash. Chowkhamba Krishnadas Academy, 2015.

Bensky, Dan, Steven Clavey, Erick Stöger, and Andrew Gamble. *Chinese Herbal Medicine: Materia Medica*. Eastland Press, 2004.

Deadman, Peter. *A Manual of Acupuncture*. Journal of Chinese Medicine Publications, 2007.

Goldstein, Joseph. *Mindfulness: A Practical Guide to Awakening*. Sounds True, 2013.

Hanna, Thomas. *Somatics*. Da Capo Press, 1988.

Hartranft, Chip. *The Yoga-Sutra of Patañjali: A New Translation with Commentary*. Shambhala Publications, 2003.

Jarrett, Lonny S. *Nourishing Destiny*. Spirit Path Press, 2004.

Juhan, Deane. *Job's Body*. Station Hill Press, 1987.

Maciocia, Giovanni. *The Foundations of Chinese Medicine: A Comprehensive Text for Acupuncturists and Herbalists*. Elsevier Churchill Livingstone, 2005.

Muktibodhananda, Swami. *Hatha Yoga Pradipika*. Yoga Publications Trust, 1993.

Myers, Tom. *Anatomy Trains*. Churchill Livingstone, 2001.

Netter, Frank. *Atlas of Human Anatomy*. Saunders, 2023.

Pitchford, Paul. *Healing with Whole Foods*. North Atlantic Books, 2002.

Rochat de la Vallée, Elisabeth. *Aspects of Spirit*. Monkey Press, 2013.

Scheid, Volker, Dan Bensky, Andrew Ellis, and Randall Barolet. *Chinese Herbal Medicine: Formulas & Strategies*. Eastland Press, 2009.

Svoboda, Robert, Arnie Lad. *Tao and Dharma: Chinese Medicine and Ayurveda*. Lotus Press, 1995.

Unschuld, Paul U. *Huang Di Nei Jing Ling Shu: The Ancient Classic on Needle Therapy*. University of California Press, 2016.

Unschuld, Paul U., Hermann Tessenow, and Zheng Jinsheng. *Huang Di Nei Jing Su Wen: An Annotated Translation of Huang Di's Inner Classic—Basic Questions*. University of California Press, 2011.

INDEX

ABOUT THE AUTHOR

Jennifer Raye is an internationally recognized Chinese Medicine practitioner and yoga and meditation teacher. She holds a doctorate in Traditional Chinese Medicine with professional licensure in acupuncture and herbal medicine.

Jennifer's unique approach, which resonates with a diverse range of students, reflects her comprehensive formal training and extensive clinical and teaching experience. Her work is a holistic and integrative blend of Chinese Medicine, yoga, meditation, Ayurveda, holistic nutrition, somatic studies, and therapeutic movement. Classes and programs with Jennifer weave physical remedies and practices with contemplative awareness as well as philosophical, energetic, and anatomical teachings.

In addition to writing and maintaining her private medical practice, Jennifer teaches workshops, retreats, and teacher training courses online and in person. She is the founder of the Inner Path Institute, an online school offering education, inspiration, and guidance in holistic healing and the meditative arts. Jennifer is grateful to live and work nestled in the mountains and forest of British Columbia, Canada. Learn more at jenniferraye.com.